ADVANCE REVIEWS

"Social Media meets Cancer (and Social Media triumphs!). This book compiles the real-time emails of Meg Stafford as she keeps her network of friends 'abreast' of her progress through the diagnosis and successful treatment for breast cancer. Without self-pity or self-absorption (she keeps working as a clinical counselor despite everything that is going on in her life), Meg details her very personal impressions and emotions of the impact of cancer. No matter how close you may have been to cancer in your life, I am certain that this book will resonate with the most fundamental notions of friends, family, and self. Meg has a remarkable ability to encapsulate the moment, no matter how small or large, in nuggets of witty wordplay that show the resiliency of her spirit and the importance of community in supporting a person through the challenges of illness and intensive therapy aimed at cure. This book should be required reading for medical students, physicians and care-givers who want to learn more about what is going on inside the head of a patient facing cancer. In a world of instant information, Meg's thoughtful descriptions of her path keep us mindful of the power of individual experience and the impact of family, community and care-givers."

— George D. Demetri, MD, Director, Ludwig Center at
Dana-Farber/Harvard Cancer Center

"With bare honesty, humor and a sparkling heart, Meg courageously extends her hand and engages in the conversation of life. Like listening to the story of a dear friend for the first time, the reader is moved to tears, delighted in muse, and inspired to reach within to gain strength and courage to live life a new way. This beautifully written memoir is an empowering and contagious illustration of the richness and possi-bility that unfold when listening to one's own voice and living each day consciously. Relevant and remarkable for anyone whose life is impacted by waves of uncertainty or personal struggle, *Topic of Cancer* is an invaluable reminder that, in the face of life's most challenging journeys, we are not alone."

— Colleen, 38-year-old husband has been dealing
with disabling cardiac disease

"Tears came at unexpected times and just as quickly went away as Meg Stafford provided what I had longed for during my sister's cancer treatment—information that could be understood by both my head and my heart. I gratefully took in information from Meg that my sister's doctors either weren't inclined to provide or perhaps weren't even aware would be welcomed. I finally felt that cancer treatment had been de-mystified. The 'Aha! Take-Away' from Meg Stafford's book: TREATMENT CHOICES. If you assume you have them, you will. For me, the essence of this book is said best by Meg herself. 'He (the doctor) asked whether I felt that I was able to resume my life. I told him that I had never stopped living it.'"

— Kate Gilligan, lost her sister to lung cancer.

To Phyllis & Jim,

May the waves you ride
bring in a tide of joy.

with love,
Meg

Topic of Cancer

Riding
the
Waves
of the Big C

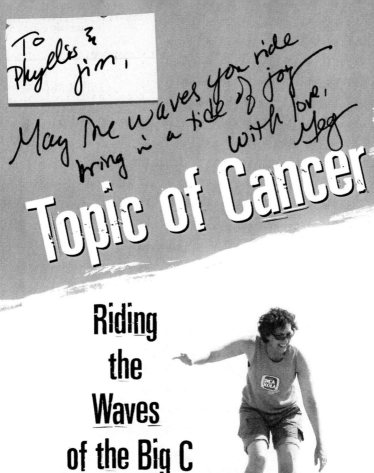

Meg Stafford

Virginia Martin Press

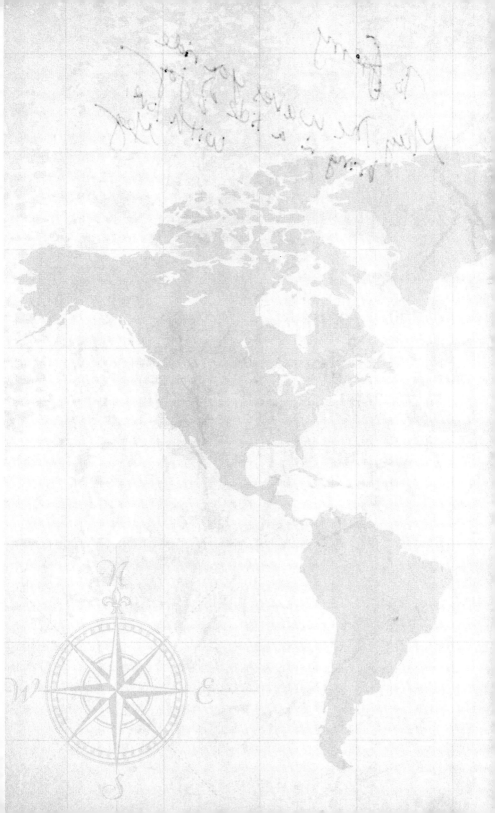

"My mission in life is not merely to survive, but to thrive; and to do so with some passion, some compassion, some humor, and some style."

— Maya Angelou

Topic of Cancer: Riding the Waves of the Big C
by Meg Stafford

ISBN: 978-1-936214-36-5

Library of Congress Control Number: 2010940428

Published by Virgina Martin Press
A Wyatt-MacKenzie Imprint

Table of Contents

Introduction

I have been trying to figure out what my relationship is to the word "survivor". Apart from the way it makes me think of the champions of the now-iconic TV show, why does it niggle at me so?

Where is the discomfort for me? What is the part of "survivor" that doesn't fit? In the midst of many positive words that can be associated with it—strong, resilient, tough, persistent, patient—what is my hesitation?

Perhaps it is that I also associate survival with natural disasters or abuse of some kind. Maybe I feel that in order to be a survivor, one must first have been a victim, and I do not want to identify with that. I always felt I had choices. With the consultation of my medical team, I could sift through which treatments I felt were most appropriate, and in what order. I believe this was a key to why I could not adopt the victim stance. I was afforded options and decisions at every turn. Even if I felt burdened by them, without sufficient knowledge or time to make them, they were still mine to make and my family and friends backed me every time.

I might have made different choices at another time in my life, if my children were younger, or older, or if I were not living so near outstanding medical help, or if I did not have the unfailing support of my husband, family and friends—my Breasty Business team, as I called them. Each person must make his or her own decisions about what is enough or too much, and no one else can know what that feels like. As consumers of medical care, as patients, it is our job to pay attention to the information given to us, and also to what our own responses and feelings are. We must make our choices from a position of strength in knowing who we are.

Perhaps, too, I am reluctant to take on the mantle of "survivorship," feeling that I did no more than live day to day, dealing with each issue as it came up. It was not about "getting through." At any given time, I could enjoy the cat leaping into the air, or the bloom of the trees, or I could feel the pain of another person's disappointments. It was about feeling it all, being present with what is, the what is of each day. "Survivor" can feel like too grand a term, too big. And yet when all those days are stitched together, at the end of treatment, I have moved from being a person undergoing treatment to one who has finished the bulk of it. Hence, the shift to survivor.

So if survivor doesn't fit, exactly, what does? I thought about thrivor, and although I like the upbeat quality of this, it is still in response to survivor, an alternative based in the surviving mode. Not quite right.

Victor? Although many people do use terms like battling cancer, and this image might work well for them, it feels too edgy, too angry. Although I needed to harness an aggressive stance, I cannot get my arms around what I perceive to be the anger to "do battle."

What about learner? Perhaps one of the biggest lessons for me during my triathlon of treatment was in how to let other people help me. People who know me well will tell you that I am a tad independent, a tiny bit stubborn, and just a wee bit tenacious in my approach. So how was I going to respond to offers of food, rides, books, clothing, or help round the house? I would always do whatever I could myself, despite people's advice to milk this time for what it was worth. I preferred to drag the laundry basket downstairs myself in my attempts to feel "normal." But I could not drive myself to chemotherapy, not with the

IV Benedryl which preceded some of the toxins, zoning me out completely. And although usually on the active side (some might say hyper), there were days when I could only do my sloth imitation.

I learned that despite my fears about being a burden, people were not only willing to help, but happy to do so. And every morsel of food delivered, every positive thought sent my way helped to relieve my own struggles, helped to diffuse the intensity of being treated for breast cancer. I'm a communicator , and I sent out messages on my Breasty Business e-mail distribution list, and people were willing to listen, willing to hear my ramblings, my rants, my musings and discoveries and assuage my pain from all corners of the globe. Although I may have feared that accepting help would make me feel "weak" or "victimized," this was not the case.

If the opposite of fear is love, I drew strength from my team to squeeze out the fears. By focusing on the gifts that other people offered, I learned about how others can be present, thoughtful, available, and giving, time and time again. How can I use the term "survivor" in the face of this kind of generosity?

On the other hand, how can I not? How can I turn away from this title, hard earned and actively addressed?

It is the strength of humans' love for one another that is helping to overcome the fears engendered by cancer. Although I am still not sure what the best term is, there are more of us now to talk about our experiences, who have survived; as we go forward, those numbers will swell, until people don't even remember what cancer was, and this little dilemma about what to call those of us who have been treated for it will be a thing of the past.

Chapter 1

The Changing Landscape

On Memorial Day 2007, I returned from my 20-mile biking loop on Cape Cod and discovered that the landscape of my chest had changed. A new foothill had developed in the usual mountain range, close to the middle of my body. It was not painful, except to my eye, as it had appeared unbidden. I called my primary care physician the next day and made an appointment for the day after.

She was unconcerned, given its quick presentation and the way it felt to her physically, but encouraged me to schedule a mammogram and ultrasound. She warned me to be prepared for the possibility of what was likely a cyst being lanced right then during the ultrasound.

A couple of weeks later I found myself in the waiting room, on deck for the ultrasound. A woman walked by who I knew years before, from our children's music class. She obviously worked there and greeted me, then didn't know quite what to say. People do not get ultrasounds as a way to build more relaxation into their lives. "Nice to see you," was about the depth of what we could exchange.

The ultrasound confirmed what the mammogram had shown: a mass that was not a cyst. I needed to schedule a biopsy. This was routine and still not cause for huge concern, as the vast majority of these are benign. Nonetheless, time went into that oddly warped pattern where days expand into centuries, and my sense of urgency was not matched by that of the medical system, which has its own schedule and priorities.

My husband, Duke, and I had not included other people in the knowledge of this process, but felt that it was now time to bring them on board, as it has always been my belief that sooner is better than later when telling people about medical stuff. There is rarely an advantage to waiting, even for the teller. Thoughts and feelings expand in the interim, giving more charge and weight than are necessary, certainly more than are helpful. If there is difficult news, most people are appreciative of being told early on, as this conveys, "You can handle this; I know you can. I care about you, and want to include you in this important aspect of my life." When too much time has passed, people can hear, "You could not handle this," or worse "You are not important enough to discuss this with."

With still not much news, we told immediate family that I was having a biopsy, that no one was sounding any alarms, and that we would have the results in a few days.

Duke and I scheduled a meeting with the surgeon to talk about possibilities. Some medical systems will not have you meet with a surgeon until the results of a biopsy are in. Others prefer to have you meet with the surgeon in advance so that, in case there is further treatment, at least some contact has been made. Ours is the latter variety. In her no-nonsense way, our petite firecracker of a surgeon laid out the tree of options. She was clear, direct, and patient, at once assuming that we understood what she was saying but that we would not get it all the first time around. My husband and I had joked beforehand about this meeting being a terrible excuse to have a mid-week date.

Afterward, we sat stunned by the graphicness of the possibilities: dissection of one lymph node plus removal of the known lump, or complete lymph node dissection if any cancerous cells were found in the sentinel node (nearest the lump) during the lumpectomy. We agreed that this was categorically the worst date we had ever been on.

She would call us a few days later with the results of the biopsy. I received the call at work, a singularly bad place to take this call, as obscenities emitting from the office of a psychotherapist, by the therapist, are not generally regarded as a great recommendation for that practitioner. So I held it together until I got home, where I was greeted and surrounded by Duke and Gale, our eldest daughter who is sweet, sassy, and 17. Kate, our 12-year-old who is sweet, sassy in her own way, and just a bit shy, had not been at home when I had called to warn them, and this was a difficult moment for her, as she saw our embrace but hadn't yet been clued in. We told her right away, but I was to learn later that even those few moments of not knowing the situation were difficult, confusing, and anxiety provoking. We did not do this again, as we made an effort to keep the girls in the loop at all times, for their sakes as well as ours. We needed each other. Our strength as a family would be challenged, but there was never a question about whether we could do it; it was always about how it would be best.

As we began to make calls to friends and family, it became clear that as important as it is to keep people informed, the process of updating everyone individually would be too cumbersome. What resulted was an e-mail distribution list that from the beginning I called the Breasty Business Update. The people on the list have been my Team, my resource, and the Update has been a permeable membrane of expression and correspondence. It has been packed with all the drama, frivolity, and tenderness that characterized my experience.

More than one person has remarked that the Update has helped them to understand some other family member who has had a similar experience. Others have declared that should they need to go through a similar experience, they now felt it would be possible. Their encouragement has inspired this quest to edit the Breasty Business Update into a form from which other people can glean what they will. Glean on me.

My in-laws happened to visit the weekend after my lumpectomy, while I was awaiting word from the pathology report. My mother-in-law had been diagnosed two years earlier with multiple myeloma and had been taking various poisons in the hope of staving off the disease's hold. It turned out that she, too, was waiting for results from a test to see whether that particular round of chemo was effective. "So we're both waiting for results," she observed. Cancer is an odd way to forge a new bond, one neither of us would ever have imagined. As soon as she uttered the words, however, my heart sank. I had the immediate sense that neither of us would have good news, but hers would be worse. Uncannily, this proved to be exactly the case. While my positive biopsy brought confirmation of breast cancer, there were ready treatments. Her levels were growing despite the metals, and as I headed toward my own chemotherapy, she was heading into the last months of her life. It was not evident at first, but the deeper into the fall we went, the more obvious it became.

The lumpectomy was scheduled for July 6. I took my last bike ride of that summer on July 4, enjoying my favorite loop through the Harvard hills, which affords the best panorama around.

July 12, 2007
The Only Way Out Is Through

Okay, so the blip is growing in size. The good news is that the rest of the 14 lymph nodes were clear. And that really is good news. The bad news is that there were cancer cells in the breast tissue surrounding the lymph nodes. This is away from the lump that was removed, so my surgeon is recommending mastectomy. It is not unusual for lobular invasive breast cancer (the type that showed up) to present in multiple sites, but nonetheless its very name sounds scary. Invasive. An intruder. Resciniti, my surgeon, is away next week, as is the plastic surgeon (have you ever met a surgeon made of plastic?), and I have appointments with both of them for the week following. I also have a marker that may put my other breast at risk, so should we go for the double deal? And what about chemotherapy?

These are all questions that we can address with the two consults we have set up for Monday. Susan, my dear internist friend, offered to accompany us to both. Her husband, a prominent physician at Dana Farber, helped us set up the consult there. We're reeling, but trying to steady ourselves for the next round of input, and treatment. Sucks. Can I just say that one more time? SUCKS!!! Duke and I were talking last night, and though my breasts have served me well, it may be time to part ways. (Duke was reminded of the John Wayne movie, True Grit, where his horse gets shot out from under him, and he says something about never having reason to doubt his horse, but that the time had come to go their own ways.)

Still, most of my tears come from the generosity of everyone receiving this, and some who haven't. There has never been any doubt about the wonderfulness of the people surrounding me, but to have it demonstrated already in such graphic ways moves me on a daily basis.

I couldn't face another round of calls, but I'm happy to hear from you, by phone or e-mail, whichever suits. I'm trying my best to not move around a lot, rather a large challenge for someone who needs several hours of biking or swimming every week in order to be happy sitting still. My goal of the week is to get this flipping drain out. It's a tube that's stitched into the under arm lymph node area to provide an exit for the excess fluid resulting from the dissections. It's more uncomfortable than anything else, and I'm likely looking at another round of the drain game, so time off from it will be welcome.

I think I'm starting to babble, and I can't even blame it on the Vicodin. Damn! I'll update again once there's more to report. I have taken to wearing Duke's button-down, easy to put on and take off, roomy shirts. "Duke Couture," I'm calling it.

Mid July 2007

Sometimes it is the smaller moments between the larger, dramatic ones that define the contrast, and highlight what is happening.

In between 3-hour-long consults at the Dana Farber and Emerson

Hospitals, we revived ourselves with sustenance at "Not My Average Joe's", as my friend's 8-year-old calls it, and then stopped at the post office to mail to Kate, our 12-year-old, the rubber bands for her braces and a phone card to have at camp. I hopped out of the car and was pleased to see only two people in line ahead of me, plus the woman at the window who was mailing a package. The post-master was stamping the woman's package with a denotation that was too small and too far away for me to read. I realized that he was covering it in stamps, easily 9 or 10 times per side of the box. He was like a child with a new stamper, trying it out, experimenting, each time delighting in the mark that it made. The repetition was mesmerizing, if a little confusing.

At some point, he must have asked the woman whether she wanted to send it registered mail, because he launched into a monologue about how good it is.

"If I die," he said gravely, "and I send my remains to my family, I will send the package by registered mail. They might get it and say, 'Oh, he must have gained some weight. This is heavy.'" As our brows furrowed and our jaws gave in to gravity, he continued, "One time we got a package through here, and boy it was heavy. That must have been some big guy." At this point, he was cutting the form to exactly match the shape of the box. The woman whose package so captivated him glanced furtively back at the growing line of customers, and I started looking around for Rod Serling. I didn't see him right off the bat, but he had to be lurking somewhere in the back.

The guys in front of me each wanted one book of stamps—$8.40 for the Cracked Bells, they were informed, and much more if the bells were whole. Then it was my turn. I feared some type of strange interaction and all I wanted was to get my package to Kate as quickly as I could and to get out of there. Whew! I was able to do this successfully. Still, Duke wondered what had taken so long, and we both hurried home to rest before the next conference.

Two days later, I had my annual physical with my internist. I was checking in at the front desk.

"Do you have your insurance card?" the receptionist asked.

"I do, but I was just here, and you took a photocopy then, I think."

"Oh, you're right," she says after checking my chart. "No change of address or phone? No drama since then?"

"Oh yes," I assured her. "There has been drama."

"No adventures?"

"Yes, there have been plenty of adventures, too," I tell her. But I had been able to achieve all that without changing my address or phone. Imagine.

I'm taken into a room where a tech takes my pulse and temperature. She's about to take my blood pressure, and has a quick form to fill out.

Any chance that you're pregnant?

No, definitely not.

Any chemotherapy or radiation?

"Not yet," I reply.

She smiles. "A patient with a sense of humor," I can tell she is thinking.

Am I living in a parallel universe here? Perhaps Rod has switched his address from post to medical office. I'm not sticking around to find out, though. I'm going back to the familiarity of my own personal limboland.

July 16, 2007
Cocktails for One

There are only a couple of definitive things that I can tell you about today. The rest will have to wait until we get more info from the slides and pathology, probably by Tuesday of next week.

First of all, the drain is gone! The drain of my existence, removed! I saw the on-call surgeon because I was concerned about some swelling, but it must have been swollen with pride because the fluid that had been collecting seems to have receded somewhat. Whew! Glory Be!

The other thing we can count on is chemotherapy. Heavy metal, here I come. Never had much of an affinity before, but it's time to start. Not sure what mix, but it'll be a blend of a certain few. They agreed on that. There will be more surgery, but it's not clear what until all the news is elicited from the report. What exactly is going on with those cells that were near the lymph nodes and away from the lump? Are the other nodes actually clear? The slides will be scrutinized more closely, reviewed by the Tumor Board (there must be a better name for that group), and I will hear back from Dana Farber (Dr. Partridge) on Tuesday of next week. Emerson (Dr. Dubois) hopes to have more info in a few days.

Dana Farber leans toward chemo first. Emerson leans toward surgery first. The order is not critical, and they will talk and come up with a plan. The hospitals are, in fact, affiliated. Both docs are lovely people, very knowledgeable about the field, and both emphasized the terrific outlook in terms of prognosis. They also both noted my stellar support system, and commented on the importance of this for recovery. Cancer is a tough thing for someone who is alone. My biggest fear is that I will have everyone snoozing by the time they get to the end of a missive.

The other good news is that I have hormone receptors, which means that this will be the last part of my treatment which will go on for a long time, and bodes the best in terms of the long-term picture. It will likely be Tamoxifen, taken as a daily pill. I also have negative HerTu (her, too? Hurt, ooh?), which is a good thing. And the aggressiveness of the tumor is moderate, which is also good. The fact that I exercise is in my favor, as is the fact that the chemo will likely put me into menopause, as for some reason, that means I will get better benefit from the treatment. It's a normal time for me to be heading there anyway. This is brought to you in rather primitive terms. Susan, my generous internist bud, was there at both consults, doing the marathon day (three hours at Dana Farber, over two at Emerson). I will be followed by an oncologist on an ongoing basis; good thing I'm not paranoid, or this could present problems.

I get misty at unexpected times and I get frustrated at certain things I can't do; I can't lift heavy things. I can't swim or bike or carry a simple load of groceries. It makes me crazy to have everyone going through this. At the same time that I am profoundly grateful that each member of my family has support from elsewhere, it makes me wild that I cannot be the one who is there all the time. I cannot calculate the toll it takes on each of us, and in what ways.

Your generosity continues to blow me away in terms of rides, food, books, flowers, checking in, willingness to listen to me ramble when I talk, and willingness to read when I ramble on screen. This is a long wave we got here, and I will do my best to ride it. Just putting some finishing touches on my surfboard and cranking up the tunes.

I love you all, and must sign off before the computer booger gets greedy with my words. More soon.

July 22, 2007
Hello, Dolly

So my left breast has decided to enter a contest with Dolly Parton. This is not a decision I endorse or approve of in any way. Neither does my right breast, which is left out of this competition, and knows that they're supposed to be a team. My left breast has accomplished its entry requirements by hoarding old blood from the lumpectomy, creating a large, gelatinous hematoma that cannot be drained by ordinary aspiration methods with a needle, or even with the guidance of ultrasound. I know this because in my efforts to thwart this enterprise I have met with Dr. Cahill, the on-call surgeon, several times this week and we have tried these interventions to no avail. There is too much there for it to be absorbed, which is what the body usually does with a hematoma.

She recommended not drinking or eating after midnight to allow the possibility of proceeding with a surgical intervention (when the hematoma will be evacuated) tomorrow afternoon. However, in my effort to regain some shred of control here, I requested possibly waiting until after I see my own surgeon on Tuesday afternoon. This is largely because I don't want to cancel my Monday clients last minute for the THIRD time in just a few weeks. I am frustrated about disrupting everyone's visits while I deal with the demands of treatment and medical schedules. Since there is not a tremendous amount of urgency, we agreed to go with this plan. This likely works out better for my surgeon as well, since tomorrow (Monday) is her first day back from vacation. At any rate, try though my left gal might, her days as a DD cup are numbered. We just don't know which number.

They might have even tried to tuck it into my next surgery, but that won't be for at least a few weeks, as I'm waiting for the results of my genetic testing, and I will hopefully start chemo anyway. Still, this charade has gone on long enough. It is not comfortable to hang around waiting for her to realize that, try though she might, she really cannot compete with Dolly. So I'm looking forward to Evacuation Day, sometime this week.

Stay tuned!

July 23, 2007
Goodbye, Dolly

The plan for Dolly's deflation is for Wednesday afternoon at two. I plan to be home by five, eating something delicious (like a rip roarin' salad) because I will not have eaten all day. I want you all to know that I have actually cancelled my meeting for Wednesday morning, instead of moving it to 8 a.m. and then just cruising into the hospital for my noon check in. How's that for some serious limit setting?

Tomorrow is information day: two appointments with surgeons and a call from the Dana Farber oncologist. I will write when coherence returns.

July 25, 2007
Stump the Surgeon

Let's play stump the surgeon. We're in the surgeon's office, reading his diploma for the fifth time, when my cell phone rings. It's Ann

Partridge, the oncologist from Dana Farber. I'm worried that we will be interrupted by the surgeon, but we continue. The Board met, and they definitely recommend mastectomy, as invasive cells were found in two other areas besides the lump area. She still presents the same choices as far as chemo, basically a cocktail of two or three chemicals, or the trial which would involve not knowing whether I was receiving a new medication. I try to press her about her recommendation, but it seems that if I don't participate in the trial, she would recommend the standard of care right now, or Adriamycin Cytocin for four treatments. She does not recommend a 2-for-1 sale (in terms of breast removal) at this point, to be revisited after we get the results of the genetic testing in a couple of weeks. I ask about the safety of the other breast, given that these other cells did not show up on MRI, but she reiterates her recommendation. Okay, so not a lot new, but confirmation that Dolly's days are, indeed, numbered.

The surgeon (plastic) arrives, and begins to talk reconstruction options. He has one picture of the simpler option, the implant, and any number of the more complicated, more aesthetically real-looking option: the flap, where some stomach muscle is used, and the skin from the breast is retained. He clearly prefers this option, even though it is more extensive, a much longer surgery, a week in the hospital, and a few months of recovery. He urges me to think about the big picture, and how I'll feel a few years down the road, not just during the few months of discomfort. I *am* a big picture person, but I'm thinking about both the immediate consequences of the more extensive surgery as well as what it will be like for me to be down one abdominal muscle (abominable muscle?!).

He goes on to say that most women won't miss one of these muscles unless they're professional athletes. While I am not a professional athlete, I am more than a casual exerciser. During biking months I'm out there at least 3-4 times a week, doing 20 miles each time on average. During the summer, I'm swimming 40 minutes on the days I'm not biking and sometimes on the days that I am. So I'm fond of those muscles. It appears that staying in shape is edging out the appearance of my breast on my priority list.

Next, he does an exam.

"Hm," he says. "You don't have a lot of tissue in your abdominal area. It would probably take both of the stomach muscles to create a breast similar to the other one."

When we're back in the office, Duke offers some of his muscle. The surgeon declines. When we revisit the implant idea, he says that it is not a good option if there will be radiation, because the quality of the skin suffers, and he quotes a statistic that 50 percent of implant procedures run into problems in these circumstances. He admits that he needs to consider all this, and will get back to me. I appreciate that at least he is being honest, especially in light of his obvious preference for the flap.

Next, we head down three flights to my non-plastic surgeon's office, where she takes one peek at Dolly, says "lovely," and we go back to her office for a few minutes where she explains that Dolly's deflation will take only about 20 minutes. Back into the incision from the lumpectomy, vacuum it out, and sew me back up. So that's later today.

Then, down another two flights to the radiation oncologist to make another appointment. There is a lot more information to gather before the final surgery choice is made.

So the upshot is, Dolly goes, and chemo is 90 percent certainly first, while I'm getting a second opinion about the reconstruction possibilities, radiation necessity, and genetics testing results. In the meantime, I'm making additional appointments with the wig place and acupuncture consultation, both to help cope with the side effects of my heavy metal education. All in all, an exhausting afternoon, leading to more questions than answers; but each consultation brings me some information, even if that only means finding out the right questions to ask. Let's hope this afternoon's procedure is quick and simple. It's a cruel thing to have me sitting here all morning with no food. At least I haven't decided to mow the lawn.

July 25, 2007
Evacuation Complete!

The term we coined to describe how I am about now is "vicadinny". They gave me one after the evacuation, and there is no pain, just a little loopiosity. So you'll forgive me if this is a bit looser than usual. Is that really possible, you ask? Oh yes, I answer. Just stay tuned.

The cruelest part about today was the fact that I did not get taken for my little procedure until after 4:30. This means that my stupid plastic bracelet was starting to look like a meal, as was Duke's forearm. It gave new meaning to devouring my book. Worse, Duke and my dear friend Ana, who had come to keep us company, seemed unable to keep the conversation off food. I would enjoy it and then suddenly realize that I was sucking on my gown strings (not really). Anyway, the procedure went well, and when we arrived home at 7:45, there was a meal waiting of chicken salad, bean salad, and pizza, all of which were incredibly delicious. Thank you!!

I feel no pain right now, and Dolly is wrapped to a fare-thee-well (if you'll Parton the expression) to make sure this doesn't happen again. I'm also finding that I have greater movement in my left arm. That could be the Vicodin talking, or it could be that Dolly's expansion had pressed on some nerves, making it more painful to move my arm (hell of a nerve). I'll know better in the morning, but it's encouraging nonetheless.

I'm glad to have one more step behind me. I did make about 47,000 appointments today, to gather the info for the next steps. One of them includes an appointment with our (and when I say our, I mean that in the teamly sense) oncologist, and I expect to have a plan at the end of that. I also expect that I will start chemo the week after. Now there's something to look forward to.

So, listen: one idea that I'm floating is for lots of you to wear bandanas or headscarves or hats in solidarity once my hair heads for the hills. What do you think? Is this selfish?

I'm getting called to watch our family summer show *So You Think You Can Dance*, so I will end my ramble, with promises of more once it becomes disclosed. Thank you for your messages, your love and support, and for being My Team!

July 27, 2007
After the Uniboober Day

The ace wrap is what qualified me for this quirky term.

I did work most of the day yesterday (11-6), crazy coot that I am. Yesterday marked a brief return to Duke Couture, which some of you might remember, for the post-surgical set. Back then (lo many days ago) it was a brightly colored button-down shirt and boxers. For work, it was the hot pink shirt with dark blue sailfish printed all over it, along with straight-leg khaki pants instead of boxers. The boxers were not so good for work. Today, back to my own stuff.

I am now awaiting next week's round of appointments. Such a schedule, I'm telling you.

Post Dolly's Deflation

I had no idea that beneath the large ace bandage lay so many layers of tears. It was the end of the day, and I had underestimated the toll of the workday, plus I had not expected to be coming around from general anesthesia (and his colonel Vicodin). The relief from having the wrap off brought one layer, plus getting my first visual of the size of the pressure bandage it was holding in place. Being able to breathe freely again, and realizing I hadn't been, brought another layer.

As I slowly peeled back the adhesive, I could not control the sobs. I was not ready for a surprise. I was tired from all this attention and discomfort for poor Dolly. Duke held me gently and rubbed my back, unflustered and patient.

"I was wondering when this would happen," he said softly. "You had to let go sometime."

His softness and complete acceptance brought on another round of tears.

"Does it hurt a lot?" he asked.

It didn't actually hurt at all; it was fatigue and anticipation, mixed with PMS (I found out today). He waited as little by little I peeled back the adhesive, taking with it numerous layers of gauze until just the last square lay covering what I assumed to be the sutures from the incision.

I paused, catching my breath, certain that a fresh flood lay waiting underneath that thin square of white. I asked Duke to rub my left arm, which is now often numb, or sometimes burning. Again, he tenderly massaged the insulted parts, reviving them, and my spirits along with them. I felt my breath slow down and become more even.

"Okay, I think I'm ready." I tugged at the gauze, and it gave way without much protest, exposing Technicolor Dolly, but without the enormous amount of swelling that had distorted her before. The almost normal appearance was the biggest shock, relative to previous days. It was the closest I had come to my pre-surgical self. Again, not a lot of pain, but I knew that beneath her improved exterior she was still diseased. I am glad of a few more months before her final evacuation. I was spent, but I also felt a deeper relief that could only have been released through the salty stream falling on Duke's steady, broad shoulder.

July 30, 2007
Port of Call

We seem to have determined a couple of things today. One is that chemotherapy is indeed the first of the treatments. One from Column A. The second is that we will start with the standard, tried treatment, AC (cocktail of Adriamycin and Cytocin). There will be four of these, and they will likely be spaced every three weeks, mostly by my preference. A newer way of administrating this is every other week (or dose dense), with a booster to get the white blood cell count up enough to receive it. The dose dense gets it over with more quickly, but I personally prefer to let my body recoup more before receiving the next dose. I know it will protract the amount of time I'm wig bound, but so be it. In the overall scheme of my life, it's two months, at most. So there you have it. This may well be followed by the same spacing of T (Taxol), thus potentially meaning a 24-week period during which I am receiving this treatment. We'll reevaluate after the AC.

The docs think that while this may be a bit of overtreatment for my level of disease, it is also the standard of care, and the best that they know how to throw at it. Since I am young and strong and healthy, the thinking is, why not? (I notice that I'm not considered middle age now; it's all about my youth. Isn't that nice?) I can have no regrets looking back in a few years, and I will not wonder whether I should have gone whole hog. These three drugs given as a regimen are ACT, which I think is kind of fitting. Everyone wants to be able to *do* something, and so, we will ACT.

As incredibly far as medicine has come, there are still no answers to many questions, like exactly how much is enough? There isn't a way to measure whether all the disease has been eradicated after any amount of treatment, so there is no clear answer about when to stop, or what is best. That leaves room for people's personal choices about how aggressively to treat the disease. Does someone lean toward the least amount of treatment possible or the most? Is someone physically strong enough to endure it? How old is the person? How much support is in place?

While there is much that all cancer patients have in common, there is a lot that is particular to each person, and to his or her circumstances. Does someone want to keep working as much as possible, or does he or she want the quickest possible way through? Would it be better to feel sicker but for a shorter length of time, or have periods of feeling well in between? Is it more important to be treated nearest to home or to explore every option no matter the distance?

It is at once helpful and daunting to think that some of the decision making is up to the patient. While the patient may not be the most educated about the disease and treatment, everyone can have opinions about his or her own lifestyle or preferences. Like someone who makes investments for someone else, it is important to know the circumstances and goals of the person involved. By asking the right questions, the practitioner can come up with the best plan.

All this is to say that I start with the metals (and then the medals) August 8, at my request. Since Evacuation Day will then be two weeks past, this is okay with Jon Dubois, the oncologist. Between now and then I need a bone scan, a CAT scan (but no scandal), and an echocardiogram, cardiogram, cardiogram (that was the echo). Because my veins are in hiding from all the IVs I've had, and are not all that findable on a good day, I will have an access port put into my chest in order to put in and take out fluids without making me a greater pincushion than I already am. This is one procedure that will be done in vein.

I think that's it for today's antics. Tomorrow brings fresh fun. Stay tuned.

August 1, 2007
Wiggity Diggity: A Not So Hair Raising Experience

The event that I expected to produce the most hilarity did not. And I thought I would be disappointed, but I was not. It was the great wig out. Going for a wig fitting, of all odd and unprecedented happenings.

Losing one's hair is such a public thing. With all the treatments and surgery, most of it can go undetected (except maybe when Dolly was wrapped with the pressure bandage, and stood out like Mt. Rainier on a clear day). But loss of hair, now that's out there. Nothing screams cancer patient like a bald head. And I'm sure that few things are more disconcerting than having clumps of hair falling out in the shower, or onto your pillow. No one looks forward to this, and I am no exception. So I thought that going to the Wig Place would be a huge reminder of my new status, and that if we could make it silly with crazy wigs, the whole adventure might be more tolerable.

But what I found was someone to whom this was completely normal, who did this every day, all day. Fitting women for wigs was her job, and she was cheerful, respectful, and dedicated to find something that worked for me. Simple as that.

I decided to go for a look that is close to my own right now. Each of the half dozen or so wigs she brought out was okay. One was so much darker than my natural (bottled) color that it was hard to take seriously. And one was so much lighter that it, too, didn't work. Most of them just had a lot more hair than I do, so when they sat atop my own hair, they looked a little more poofy than I'm used to. But none of them would produce the "point and laugh."

Then there's the issue of natural hair versus synthetic, which is not so tremendous a difference as I anticipated, either by feel or price. I ultimately chose a synthetic wig that had a couple of features that made it appealing to me, besides the fact that it was closest to my color and amount of curliness. It weighed less than the others and will hopefully be a little less hot (don't need to start being a hothead now!). It fit well, and had a lace front, which supposedly will look more natural on my head.

There was a relief in knowing that I will have a choice about what I put on my head after my hair departs. I'm sure I'll try out hats, wraps, and even combinations, but at least when I choose, I can put on something that, in fact, is a nicer style than I can often achieve with my own hair! So, hats off to PK Walsh, where I happened to go for my fitting. And when the wig comes in next week, I go back to have it styled and trimmed in a way that suits me. We found out that it's named Orchard, so I'll have some kind of tree on my head. One of the other ones I was considering was named Betty, one Carol, and the rest just looked like a bunch of tribbles sitting on the counter.

Probably my biggest challenge will be keeping it away from the animals and making sure that they do not see fit to mark it, claw it, or otherwise personalize it for their own uses. I can just see the cats curled up inside it; they are always insistent on sniffing my head when I've come from the hairdresser. Who knows what they'll do this time!

One more piece in place (so to speak) in this wild ride.

August 1, 2007
Slight Change In Schedule

After a little tango with the scheduling gurus, the decision was made that all my tests, plus the port placement, will happen next Wednesday, with chemo to begin on Thursday. Kind of an intense couple of days, eh, what? But they're followed by a week off work, which is helpful. More soon.

August 3, 2007
Dolly's Dilemma

Dolly has made a back door run at the competition. She thought that I was complacent, and that following her evacuation last week, I would not notice that she was pilfering fluid from somewhere in order to bump start her campaign. She might have had a chance, except that somewhere along the way some of the fluid became infected. This caused some redness, which I did notice. I put this together with the fact that Tuesday night I was really exhausted and not feeling great. When I was still feeling fatigued and just not myself on Wednesday, I called the surgeon (Resciniti) and described Dolly's antics.

She prescribed an antibiotic and asked me to come in the following morning. I did this, and was greeted by her tiny cat at the doorway to the waiting room. I was the first patient of the day, and the little cat was very friendly. She even jumped up on the receptionist's chair and up through the window for a little scratch. When she (the surgeon, not the cat) saw Dolly, she asked me to lie back, and she pulled out a bunch of fluid. Foiled again, Dolly.

"I hope we don't need to go back in to deal with this," she said (the surgeon, not Dolly).

"No kidding."

Apart from being a major drag in and of itself, it would bump my schedule back, which as we all know makes me cuckoo. I have my next appointment on Tuesday if things don't get out of hand sooner, so we'll see.

August 5, 2007
What Do You Say

I have recently come across this same situation a number of times and need to come up with a truthful but relatively brief way of responding. I'm in the parking lot of the supermarket, and I see someone who I haven't seen in a really long time. She's in her car, and I'm heading into mine with Kate and her friend.

"Hey, Meg! How are you?" In this instance, I know she has seen my older daughter in the beginning of the summer.

"Has Gale told you what's going on?"

"No, she didn't mention anything."

"Well, life's been a little complicated this summer," I reply. "I'll have to call you."

And I will. At the moment I feel good. I'm happy and going about my business generally. But I'm not going to shout across the parking lot "HEY I'm starting chemo this week! How are you?"

At the time Gale saw her, we knew very little of what was happening. I talked with Duke about it. There's really no in-between. You're either dropping the bomb, or you're faking it, and neither option really appeals. We thought, well, maybe I can say, "Oh, ye know. I've got just a wee touch of the cancer. Just a little breast cancer, don't you know. Achhh. What are you gonna do…nice seeing you…."

Back at the supermarket a few days later, again with Kate, we run into the mother of one of her soccer teammates.

"Hey," she says, "How's your summer going?" Kate and I freeze.

She looks confused and says, "It's not a hard question."

Oh yes, but it is.

"Well, I've had a major medical diagnosis, so it's a little tricky. But mostly we're okay," I say cheerfully. It feels weird. We saw her at the end of the school year, and everything was obviously fine. The girls' team went to the finals of their division, and there was a party after. Both of us look just fine. I'm not hiding anything, but was the middle of the snack isle the place to bring up my breasty business?

We see her again at the checkout. She begins to apologize. "I'm sorry. I obviously asked the wrong question."

How's your summer going? Does it get any more innocuous than that? I don't think so, so I fill her in on what's been going on, and of course she understands. The checkout people, who are probably getting dribs and drabs, are looking a little horrified, but I smile and ring up my groceries. At least I haven't got a megaphone in my hand. Then she offers to help in any way that she can, including transportation if needed.

The guy at the pool store loves to razz me. He knows that I bike and swim.

"Hey, Meg, I keep expecting to see you in the paper for strongest woman in the world." Master of the hyperbole.

"Well, I've been a little waylaid this summer. I'll be back at it soon," I reply.

I pick up my chemicals and leave, feeling a little guilty that I haven't come completely clean, but that's all I can do right now. The pool's chemotherapy is so much simpler than my own.

I describe this interaction to my family and Kate says, "You're strong in a different way this summer." That was a poetic way to put it, and very generous as well. I am touched.

Back to the question of how to answer innocent small-talk queries, can I say that the summer has been unusual and eventful? That I've been writing a lot more than usual? Corresponding like mad? Adventuring like crazy? Getting out of work at every turn? It's not clear. I will have to give this consideration, see how it goes. In the meantime, I realize that every situation has its own dimensions. How well do I know the person? How much time do we have? What is my mood in the moment? There is no formulaic answer. That's just the way it goes.

August 5, 2007
Birthday Girl

What an awesome birthday party I had today, right on my 50th! Thank you thank you to everyone for helping to create the smorgasbord and for swimming, chatting and sharing my day. Although not what we envisioned for our combined 50th birthdays/20th wedding anniversary party which was to include live music and us providing the food, it was a treat to mark the occasion with all of you. I am full.

August 8, 2007
Too many appointments

My day started at 6:00 with the excitement of evacuating 14 frogs from the pool. Yes, you read that correctly. 14!! This marks a new pool record. They did their amphibian best to evade capture, jumping out of the net and back into the water, diving into deep water where I do not have the net speed to come after them. They choreographed a dance among them, sometimes floating, sometimes diving, but always managing to make me look like a fool as I charged around the pool, stabbing at the water with my long-handled skimmer. I did, of course, prevail in the end, netting the Pool's 14. Victory is sweet, but so short lived.

After six hours in my own office, I headed to Dr. Resciniti's (the surgeon) for my post-op appointment. I didn't even get to see Samantha, the cat. She (the surgeon, not the cat) took a look at Dolly and asked her nurse to get some 30-cc syringes.

She said that she doesn't usually drain the competitors this way, but does sometimes. And she occasionally puts in a drain for a while. The D word! Oh, no!

"I hate the drain," I said quietly. And I sure hope it won't be necessary.

In the meantime, she siphoned off 100 cc of fluid from the Dollster, leaving a cavity large enough to fit a pea. I'm hoping this puts the final kibosh on Dolly's designs for the competition (hasn't the deadline passed already?). It may not be a good sign that by the time I checked on her later, the divot was already filled in.

"Come back in a week," she called over her shoulder as she went out the door.

I made an appointment for two weeks, because we're actually going to the Cape for a few days next week, with the promise that if she filled up a lot in between I would call and come in before we leave.

Resciniti sent me down to the oncologist's office; she was irritated that they had scheduled Intervention Radiology to put the port in place. I was kind of touched that she felt strongly enough about a patient to feel annoyed that someone else was going to do a surgical procedure. I don't think it's personal, but more a statement about the way she feels about her patients. She wants to be the one doing the surgery. I appreciate this desire for consistency (if that's what it is). My oncologist (Dr. Dubois, or Hugs, as I start calling him because that's the unusual way he greets me and anyone who comes with me) reassures me that the Radiation people will do a fine job as well.

More conversation with him about the treatment. He agrees that AC administered every three weeks is a fine way to go. They encourage dense dose (every two weeks) for people with more lymph involvement, as it seems to have better results; but for people like me, with only one, it doesn't hold as much benefit. He has become a bit concerned that there is not a more specific protocol for a patient with a particular profile, and hopes that he and a colleague from Mass General will soon be able to put one in place. He wants to balance enough treatment without there being too much. I feel a little like we are back to square one in terms of choices, but we are at least in agreement with the current plan, and will revisit the next options as we get closer to them. I was unprepared for this conversation. I knew that he had called, but had (incorrectly) understood that it was just to check in about all the procedures for Wednesday and Thursday.

Now I am tired from revisiting the whole issue, and having questions raised. I need rest in order to hit tomorrow's adventures with some energy. At least I get to drink tonight, and again tomorrow morning. Yummy shakes, courtesy of the CT scan. Mmmm-mmmm. Citrus chalk. Everyone's favorite.

August 8, 2007
Portable Me

I did it! The tests went amazingly smoothly today. I truly felt that the staff was making particular efforts to keep everything on track (could be that they just didn't want me roaming around the hospital unchaperoned). I'm actually giving credit for this one to you guys, my Breasty Business Team. I'm sure you were sending the message to get me out quickly and easily and they could not deny.

CT scan at 7:30, injection for the bone scan right at eight o'clock. Then they were going to draw blood to get a coagulation time, but when I cringed, someone pointed out a way to get it from the IV that was in place. One less stick of the needle was good with me. One of the nurses in radiology asked what my plans were between 8 and 11, when the bone scan would take place.

"I thought I'd go dancing," is what I replied.

"Fresh," she retorted.

They were actually fine with my going out of the hospital to run errands and go home for a little while. This proved to be a terrific idea, as it was out where there is light, and I could get gas for the car, and go to the bank, and pretend that I am not going to spend the rest of the day in a windowless place.

My friend Pam picked me up at the house, and back we went.

Bone scan promptly at 11. The part you lie on is so narrow that I just fit on it if my arms are crossed in front of me. I asked what the Patriots do if they need a bone scan, and she said that they just hang over the edge.

As I lay there, I heard a colleague of the technician say that he was leaving a card for me. She explained that although the amount of radioactive substance is no danger to my family or anyone around me, it could be picked up on scans that might be done searching for terrorist activity. So they give people these cards to establish that although I might be a terror, I am not a terrorist or a threat to my country. I imagined it to be large, 8 x 11, at least, and neon orange or yellow. But no, it's a just an unassuming business card with information on it that fits neatly into my wallet. How anticlimactic.

As soon as this was finished, the technician called up to cardiology, and the woman who does the echocardiograms said that if I came right up, she would do mine immediately. Awesome. I was taken back to pregnancy days, hearing the heartbeat as she searched around the black and white pattern on the screen.

Back to radiology, and my prep for the port placement began within two minutes. I was changed, and in the room, and woozy. The surgeon must have been detained, because I surfaced and was told that he would be coming soon. Back to Versed land. I think it's poetic that this drug is spelled that way. So now I am well versed, indeed. I did resurface as they were finishing and found it rather fascinating. I asked questions from beneath the blue sheet as I was being stitched up. It wasn't painful. I couldn't see a thing, so it was the ideal combination of drugs and no graphic images of what was occurring.

I emerged spacey, and with an appetite, which I realized when my lunch came (around 4:00).

Since then, I have continued to feel better, and with more food, even better. The port gets fluids into my body without having to bother my tiny veins that are hard to find anyway. It sits completely subcutaneously, which I hadn't realized before today. I will have a matching scar on the right side to Dolly's lumpectomy scar. I'm back to babying the port side (although since it's on my right side should it be called the starboard side?!); no heavy lifting, but after a couple of weeks, I should have very little discomfort. When they need to either inject drugs, or take blood, they do so through the skin, directly into the port, my own personal boob tube. And they can administer some anesthetic cream to help with the puncture.

So, all in all, a successful day. Long. Tiring. But uneventful beyond the scheduled excitement. Tomorrow is another day.

Chapter 2

Heavy Metal

August 10, 2007
First Round Deployed

I woke up in the middle of the night on Wednesday with some post-surgical pain, and after Tylenol didn't cover it, I took half a Vicodin, which helped a lot.

When we went in for chemo on Thursday, all went smoothly. The access to the port was in place, so the nurse just started dripping chemicals in. First came the anti-nausea drug, then the heavy hitters. I chose a pleasant, sunlit room. One other woman was there, who seemed calm and good natured. She was also a first-timer. The nurse offered lovely quilts that were donated by the Women's Auxiliary. I love quilts and picked out a very colorful winner to take home. How nice is that?

We were finished by around noon. I fell asleep on the way home, discovered more food had been dropped off courtesy of Mom, sampled some, and felt a little livelier. I needed to keep ice on the port to help keep me comfortable. It was an invaluable conduit of the chemotherapy into my system but it came with a bumpy reminder of its presence on my chest. In the afternoon, I fell asleep trying to read. I almost never nap. When I woke up, I didn't feel 100 percent—not terrible, just not totally myself.

I hit a similar wall both other times when I was a day out from surgery. Must be something about the anesthesia leaving my body, but I become intensely emotional. Any little thing can make me cry, and this time, those same things would make me laugh because I realized how absolutely absurd they were. The mercurial nature of this process was exhausting. I couldn't keep up with my own ups and downs.

This was a tad confusing for Gale and Duke, who didn't know how to react to me, or what to do. That, too, made me teary, and then it was a riot to see the expressions on their faces. I asked Duke for tissues, so he brought up a few boxes from the basement. I could see that he was moving the brown box out of the way in order to get to the blue one, which he knew I would like better. But I wanted the yellow one. It made me teary to see Duke making such an effort, knowing what I would want, and then it made me giggle because the whole thing was so ridiculous. This was a tissue box we were talking about! And so on it went.

There was nothing to do but ride it out, which took somewhere around an hour. I would try to have a good cry to just get it over with, but the idea of forcing myself to do that tickled me. Eventually, I'd return to myself. It is so weird going through these moments, but at least I have my previous experiences to know that they're time limited.

Today is another day, and we'll see how it goes. I took Ativan last night, which evidently has anti-nausea properties in addition to its sleep-assisting and anti-anxiety properties, for which it is better known. I feel a tad light-headed, but I need to get a lot of fluids going. The pain is less, and now I can start to think about the fun stuff we can do when we go to the Cape. We have to make the most of our few days there, which will be sandwiched in between appointments. Not so much in the swimming or biking department for me, but lots of walking and reading.

Thank you again for your comments, your support, and for the food and love that flood through this line. More soon.

August 12, 2007
Just A Little Filler

I'm day four out from chemo, and thus far today have been managing on my own without additional anti-nausea drugs. It's a tricky business; I need to pay close attention to when I'm hungry, and for what, and to make sure to eat little meals regularly. So far, so good.

I suspect the formula will change as the days go on, but as long as I'm tuning in to my body and what I need, I should be okay. My energy level has been pretty good. In fact, I need to do some more walking to burn some off.

Picked up the rug yesterday and wore it on errands on the way home. No one did the obvious point and laugh, which I took to be a good sign. Kate's and Duke's reactions were pretty similar; neither was shocked. It's a little bigger than my hair right now, partly because it's being pushed up by my own present head of hair. When it has the opportunity to lie more flatly on my head, it will look even better, I hope. It'll be weird for sure, but at least I'm prepared. Ish.

We will go to the Cape for a few days. The last time we went down, we noticed an illuminated road sign informing us:

PEED LIMIT 50 MPH
RICKLY ENFORCED

I wonder if you are aware of this charge to enforce the PEED limit, Rick, and exactly how do you enforce it? How does one achieve the PEED limit, anyway? I think it should be held up as an accomplishment, don't you?

I'm hoping that on this trip, either Rick has been relieved of his job, or that someone has seen fit to change the PEED limit, because after all, this is private business we're talking about here. I know it has nothing to do with my breasty business, but it just tickles me so to think about it; I can keep quiet no longer.

I have lots of appointments coming up: plastic surgeon, check my blood counts, MRI, check on Dolly (who has been behaving nicely, thank you), check on the port (it's amazing, but nothing too dramatic, I hope). Good to have a week off from work, at least. Hoping for a few days with the fam to relax, regroup, and have fun.

August 17, 2007
Tail of the Kite

I had what is called my Nadir visit today (This has nothing to do with Ralph, you'll be pleased to know). I hadn't given a lot of thought to the name before today. It was on my sheet of appointments, and there is one in between every chemotherapy treatment. Like the name implies, this is the low point. (I guess Nadir is more subtle than calling it "The time you're most-likely-to-feel-like shit and discomfort Day") Specifically, this refers to my white blood count, which bottoms out somewhere around the tenth day after treatment. This is technically day nine, but it's Friday, and these appointments don't occur on Saturday.

Had I thought about this more before, maybe I could have anticipated that chemo would not be a straight trajectory that starts with feeling lousy after a treatment, and then gets better and better until the next one. Intuition wants a way of trying to impose predictability in a landscape that is alien and without order. I need to learn how to ride the tail of the kite as it explores the wind currents and takes me places I didn't know existed. Attached to the tail is the phone number of my oncologist's office, along with various other medical personnel, and of course the phone numbers and e-mail of my Breasty Business Team.

Much of my focus had been about how to deal with the nausea. I was sent home with four, count 'em four, medications to combat my tendency to hurl. Three of them I was instructed to take for the first three days, and then after that I could try different things depending on level of nausea and level of side effect.

I have been learning to deal with the nausea primarily by altering my eating habits. Normally a morning person, this week I have been tired when I get up, and seem to pick up speed during the day. I decided that this may be an issue of fuel, so I'm making sure to eat earlier, and more substantive food. This translated into having leftover mango chicken for breakfast yesterday morning. And that seemed to help!

I did learn today that I'm a little anemic, so that explains some of my fatigue and yearning for protein. But generally, I've been feeling pretty well, and I'm happy to keep away from the complications of the meds. That alone is worth the vigilance of paying attention to the smallest vicissitudes of my system to make this work.

So, what do you do when you're keeping nausea at bay and you go on vacation to the Cape? You go for a boat ride, of course. Big boat that minimizes motion? You might think so, but that is for the faint of heart or levelheaded. Through the kindness of Bob, my brother-in-law, and his Patriot Boat compadres, we were arranged passage on a boat that transports a maximum of 40 passengers per trip—largely people that live in Falmouth and work on Martha's Vineyard, or vice versa.

Turns out that this was an awesome way to go, even in the morning when I had been working harder to stay even. The boat is heavy, and the motor is powerful, so passage is half the time of a larger ship. Direct and to the point: my kind of boat. And what a spectacular day on the Vineyard in between boat rides!

Returning to my medical self check, yesterday I realized that my tongue was a little sore.

"Call the doctor's office. That's on the list of things to call about," Duke said. At least one of us is paying attention.

I reported in, and the nurse called in two prescriptions to the Falmouth CVS. We're going to have to build an addition onto the house to accommodate my growing arsenal of medications.

One is a swish and spit, the other a swish and swallow. To my delight, the swish and swallow is a sweetly (bubble gum? banana?) flavored suspension, which seemed to help almost immediately. I learned today that the pain in my tongue is a result of my counts being low. The threat of thrush increases as the bacteria that is normally in my mouth realizes that the pesky white blood cells that usually keep them at bay have gone on vacation. Thrush is a delightful milky looking film that inhabits the mouth when its system is out of balance.

"Hey!" they tell each other. "Party in the mouth!" Soon there are all kinds of unusual events happening in there.

This is short-lived, because the white blood cell count rebounds, irritated at the party that has erupted in their absence. They then deliver a stern warning to the bacteria not to do this again or they will impose stricter consequences.

Today I noticed a rash on part of my chest and neck. What the hell? Has there been doubt about my rashonality? Can I now start rationalizing?

This could be a reaction to the new medication, or it could just be that I was having a little too much fun in the sun yesterday, and my increased sensitivity is responding with a little skin message.

Meanwhile, the flavored suspension has been suspended, and I have new things to try if the mouth issues do not resolve. Isn't this fun? The circuitous journey between treatments is doing its level best to keep me from growing complacent, or from taking anything for granted.

All of this is really silly, because I have long known that somewhere around day 14 out from chemo awaits CBD. Yes, I have been preparing as best as I can for Cue Ball Day, which is fast approaching. This should have been proof enough that although I am feeling generally well, with the odd symptom cropping up here and there, that the medicine is continuing to work its magic, rooting out aberrant cells and preparing hair follicles for summer cleaning. What was this nonsense about getting through the first few days and then sailing through until the next time?

I think I'll hold up a finger and try to catch the direction of the wind.

August 19, 2007
The Full Triathlon

We could not have chosen a more upbeat or colorful place to spend
the day than Provincetown. It was carnival day, and the whole town was
preparing for the signature event, the parade, which started at three
o'clock. There were chairs lining the main street at 11 a.m., when we
started our stroll, and it was not clear who was more excited—the partic-
ipants or the spectators. There was an air of excited anticipation as the
crowd grew in numbers, costumes, and extravagance.

Back home on Friday, we dumped our luggage (and the kids) and
raced back to Emerson for the Nadir appointment, followed by a visit
with the radiation oncologist, Dr. Schoenthaler (Laser Lady). She
reviewed the information that she had received already and asked about
my visit with the plastic surgeon, so we recapped the surgeries, and
Dolly's antics, and the post-chemo symptoms that had cropped up.

Laser Lady empathized with some of the complications. "It hopefully won't always go like that," she said.

"I think I'm doing well!" I replied. Truly, if I can feel as good as I do
now for most of my chemo, I'll be in good shape.

She looked at me and hesitated for just a fraction of a second. I
could sense her taking in what I had just said, and weighing it with the
information she had just compiled. She smiled, nodded her head as if
to say, "Okay I hear you, and I'm going with where you are in this
moment."

"Good!" is what she said aloud, and we moved on.

She went on to explain that she absolutely recommends radiation
post-mastectomy, citing her earlier experiences with women who didn't.
She explained some of the risks, talking about the tightness that some
women experience and the work entailed in regaining range of motion.
There's also a risk of arm edema, which is usually easily managed. I
resisted the urge to explain my understanding of armedema as the little
critters which inhabit dry places like Texas; she seemed so earnest, I just
couldn't do it. The risks to other organs is minimal, and she wanted to

make sure that I was aware of the impact on physical activity for me. Again, I appreciated her taking the time to see me as an individual, not a body with disease to be managed.

The upshot is that I am indeed in for the Triathlon of Treatment. I had expected this, but now it is confirmed. This does not include the reconstruction, which is still up in the air (probably catching a wind current), or the pre-triathlon training, which I have been doing all summer, leading up to the start of chemo. So here we are; one more piece of the puzzle dropped into place.

I cannot emphasize enough how much your support is vital and appreciated. It helps me to keep focus on the unanticipated opportunities this whole experience has afforded me. I continue to see my treatment as only a part of my current life experience, and I work to keep it as small a part as it can occupy. My family, my friends, my work, and the huge amount of fun and enjoyment I take from daily living, from visits, from movies, the outdoors, food, the animals, etc., far outweigh anything else. I know there will be times when the treatment fills up more of the frame, but I plan to take full advantage of the times it doesn't.

August 22, 2007
Day 14

As I mentioned, Day 14 is code for CBD (Cue Ball Day). For some women, this is the day the hair starts its own evacuation. And evidently, when it starts, it can happen dramatically, like waking up and finding a small critters' worth of hair decorating your pillow, or clogging the drain during a shower. So if I don't sleep or shower I should be all set, right? Each person is different, and the nurse last week reminded me that it could be several more days before the exodus.

When I spoke to the wig place today to try to set up an appointment for my buzz cut and final wig trim, it was a bit tricky, since there is no exact date that I know it will happen, even though I am at the magical Day 14 marker. The receptionist told me people often tell her that their scalp tingles just before their hair departs. How's that for a heads up? I love the idea; it's like Hair Control's way of sending a message. I'll let you know if it actually happens that way.

My friend Laura wondered whether it could happen all at once. Say, during a meeting with a client! This possibility honestly had not occurred to me. I'm sure as hell hoping that it's not like pressing a button and all of a sudden there's a ring of hair around me.

I can hear it now: "Hair Control to the follicles. Prepare to release, prepare to release. On my mark. Ready, set…" And then, like lemmings rushing to the sea, they would all jump at once.

This would certainly crown any past Embarrassing Moments, with clients or without. Maybe I'll bring my wig to work tomorrow, just in case.

I would be grateful to not have a hair appointment this week, as I already have three others. A visit to the surgeon yesterday yielded more drained fluid, but only a little. Today was an MRI of my liver: When a body scan is done, cysts are often found that have probably always been there, but follow-up is needed to confirm that this is the case. Friday is a consult with a second plastic surgeon. (Where do the rubber surgeons hang out?!)

But my biggest news is that I took a bike ride today! Yippee! A relatively short one for me—10 miles—but it still counts and it felt great. My biggest concern has been my left arm, which is still a bit tight. I did my best to stay away from big hills (a challenge around here), which was a good plan, because my arm did pull a little going up the small hills. I'm ready for more, particularly while it's cool and I can keep covered from the sun and still be comfortable.

I'm appreciating feeling good, and almost feeling guilty about accepting food while I'm feeling this way. Several friends and my mom have brought over food after I've had a procedure. I'm so grateful, that I'm doing away with any guilt, and just enjoying the break.

August 23, 2007
Lost My Cookies

So, I had to choose last night to lose my cookies—and the dinner that I had after them. I don't know why this happened—I'm chalking it up to my compromised immune system. One of my clients had mentioned that this kind of disgorging illness had sped through her family. Normally, I shrug off these little menaces, but in my vulnerable state, I'm guessing that I picked it up.

At 1 a.m., I thought it might be a good idea to take one of my anti-nausea meds, given that I have such a variety. Since Diet Coke was the only soda we had in the house, I chose to sip some and go with the Ativan. Oops. I forgot that I should Never Take More Than one-half of Those Wacky Little Pills. Otherwise, I'm knocked on my butt for hours. Which I was.

Fortunately, I didn't start work today until 10, which meant that I didn't have to drag myself out of bed (or couch) until after 8:30. Kate made me some coffee (with caffeine, even) which helped bring me around, and Gale made me some lunch to take with me. Off I went. I started to come around by six in the evening, and now I'm fine. So it must have been a bug. Homemade turkey soup (thanks, Peter) fixed me right up.

By the way, Duke and Gale are quite thrilled with the recent news of my slight anemia. I'm trying to boost my iron by starting to eat red meat and more spinach. Duke lost no time in bringing home steak tips, which he usually reserves for nights when Kate and I are both out. I can tell that I must need it, because it's appealing to eat it.

Before I went out for my bike ride yesterday, Gale asked me sternly what I had eaten that morning. When she learned that I had eaten a muffin and two homemade chocolate chip cookies she suggested that I have a peanut butter sandwich first. I countered with a couple pieces of steak, and she agreed to let me go if I ate those. What is the world coming to? My kids are monitoring my food, and I'm suggesting steak for snacks? Honestly.

Still waiting breathlessly for CBD.

August 26, 2007
What's the Buzz? or Visit with PS

My biggest thrill of the past few days is that I have gone swimming a couple times. It is exquisite. It is a moving meditation for me, and is helping to loosen up my arm, too. Only a few days left with our pool, so I'm trying to take advantage. It just feels great.

Visit with PS #2 (plastic surgeon, Driscoll) was Thursday. The routine was the same. First a chat in the office to discuss the options, then an exam to see which of these options is really viable, then another chat to wrap up. This one was more definitive than the last, although he was clearly a bit perplexed.

I was relaying some of the conversation to Kate, who had spontaneously come with me so that she could visit a camp friend who lives in Newton, near the doctor's office.

"You're kind of unorthodox," the doctor began.

"Ooh, good pick-up," commented Kate.

"In what way?" I asked (the doctor, I mean. I knew what Kate meant).

"Well, first, people usually do surgery first (with the reconstruction), and then chemotherapy and then radiation. You're starting with the chemotherapy, which I understand. But second, you're working with a radiation oncologist who doesn't want to irradiate with any kind of reconstruction."

The tricky part about this is that reconstruction (with tissue expander) cannot happen after radiation, because the radiation makes the skin too tight and inelastic. He agrees that although the tram flap is aesthetically the most pleasing, this is not really a great option for me. (This is the one that uses stomach muscle.) He recommends the tissue expander, to be replaced by the implant. This is a less complicated surgery, as tissue and muscle are not being moved as much. It does involve multiple surgeries, as the hard plastic tissue expander needs to be replaced by the softer implant made of silicone or saline. The first plastic surgeon had been concerned about complications doing this with radiation.

I now need to go back to Laser Lady and ask exactly what her concerns are about radiating with the expander in place. Is it that to radiate around it causes greater risk to minor little organs like my heart, or that the radiation itself is compromised because of it? I do not want to pit safety against aesthetics.

Driscoll also talked about the psychological aspect of waking from surgery and finding that, although changed, there is still something there. Instead of the loss of the body part completely, when a tissue expander is partially inflated it creates the illusion of a breast. It is a less dramatic change, already on the way to more closely mimicking the well breast. I understand this, but I have not yet decided what will work best for me.

He also mentioned a new kind of surgery that is only being done at Beth Israel and the Brigham. It's called a DIEP flap and involves tissue (usually stomach), but not muscle, and is a long (10-hour) surgery. I'm not sure this is for me, either. More research may be needed. After all, I will be down on my quota of appointments for the next couple weeks if I don't set up a few more.

I think I'll pay a visit to the gal in Fitchburg, the sister to the wig place owner, who is developing breast prostheses that are more realistic looking. Again, this may be the simplest option. Good thing I've started with the chemo so that I don't feel pressured around making the surgical decisions.

On to the hairy issues. Mine has decided to start vacating the premises.

Not in huge droves, but it's definitely gearing up for the major vacation. I've made an appointment for Tuesday afternoon to create my GI Jane look (or the Sinead O'Connor look, which has a gentler feel to it). They assure me that I should be fine until then, as I have not had the tingly thingy yet (at least not much), and I have not experienced the sudden appearance of hair on my pillow. I think it'll actually take a little while before I can truly call it CBD (absolutely no hair), but for all intents and purposes, Tuesday is the day. My plan is to wear makeup that day, and maybe a really nice dress, so that I can welcome in the new look as the special occasion that it is.

This is definitely an area where it is helpful to have some say in the matter. The hair is taking its leave, but I can choose the timing of the major alteration. It's unsettling to have clumps come out in the shower, but it is also amazing how much hair we humans have. I don't have especially thick hair, so it's just a matter of time before it starts to look patchy.

Move over, Mr. Dog, I'm shedding with the best of them now. I could make those dust bunnies you produce look puny.

Before it was clear that I would get an appointment at the wig place, where I will have a private room for the buzz, Duke offered up his barber, Priscilla Champagne, to do the job. I was imagining the guys in there, lined up for their own cuts, and me, sitting down with the big white apron, looking at the clippers, waiting for the buzz to begin. I imagined them looking on; maybe Duke could coach them in the Breasty Business cheer.

I'm not sure I'm ready for that amount of publicness. I happen to have the option of a little privacy for those first few moments. Why not take advantage? There will be plenty of time to be public, lots of drivers at stoplights to surprise if I so choose.

Gale also offered to do the job with Duke's beard-trimming clippers. This made me teary, as I appreciate her generosity but could not bear for her to have to be the one to execute this change.

It's been good to have a couple of days to get used to the idea of Cue Ball Tuesday. It has the extra advantage of being my last day of work until after Labor Day, too. I just hope I don't miss out on the tingly part!

August 28, 2007 (in the morning)
Point of Information

I'm not going! I'm not going! I'm not going! Aaaaaaaaah! But I do have on my most colorful dress, and am I ever glam on the make-up front.

Buzz on!!

Sorry about the confusion for some of you who thought that this morning's protest meant that I was canceling the appointment. I was just going back to the paratrooper's method of saying "I'm not going!" before jumping. I did, indeed, jump.

The Long and Short of It

The eagle has landed. The bald variety, that is. I trooped into PK in my hot pink rubber flip flops with the green polka dot bows and announced my arrival. Susan came a few minutes later and sat me down in the chair, asking if I would like to watch.

"I'm not sure," I replied.

"I usually start people off not watching."

She turned my chair at a little bit of an angle so that I could see a bit out of my peripheral vision, but would need to turn my head to look directly. That seemed like a good way to go. I heard the buzz that one might usually associate with the dentist's chair, and she began to clip.

In a few minutes, I turned to check out her handiwork.

"I can go shorter if you want me to," Susan said.

I would need to whip out my magnifying glass if she went any shorter.

"No, I think that's fine."

"You have a cute head," she said. "You really do."

Uh-huh.

Next, we popped on the wig. Just a little clipping on the side and I was good to go. In less than half an hour, my hair situation had been transformed to two new options.

I rode home to discover that Kate was just being dropped off by her friends, and Gale arrived a minute later. I was gathering myself, trying to regain balance, and not quite ready for contact. Both girls looked at me without much comment.

Uh-oh.

They were trying to think of something to say, I could tell. After a few minutes of puttering around, I took a deep breath and offered to show them my new look underneath the wig. Might as well dive in at the deep end.

I was surprised that they both wanted to, and both had the same reaction: "Oh, I like it! Much better than the wig."

The buzz, as different as it is, is at least mine. I like having the hair off my face. The wig looks different, and I have to admit, it is kind of hot and itchy in 85 degree weather. Well, one hurdle down. At least I don't mind the wig for when I need it, if it's not too hot.

I will have to experiment with scarves, and hats, the wig, and not. It will take a while to get used to it all. The bristles will continue to fall out, leaving me with a truly bald head at some point.

Duke called, eager to hear, and I was still trying to re-center. He could hear my hesitation and reluctance, the verge of my tears. He arrived home awhile later toting flowers, which inevitably make me smile. He is my Wizard of Vase.

I will now re-experience swimming, biking (may need something on under the helmet), and all kinds of weather. We'll see how it goes.

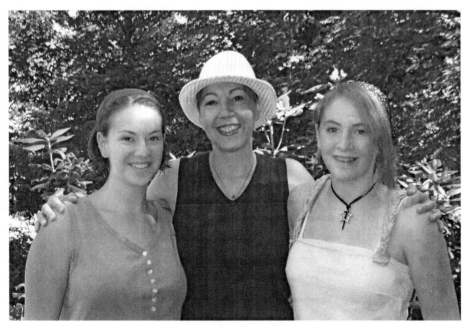

Several Days post CBD

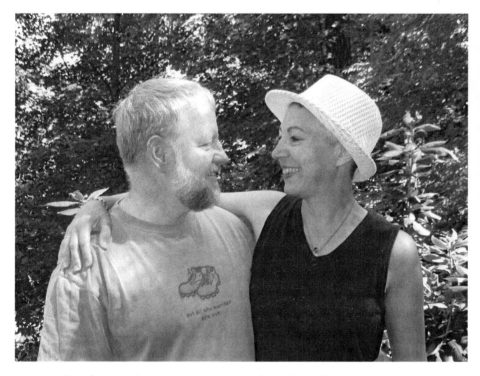

Another day, another issue to work out. Not physically strenuous, but an emotional grabber.

September 3, 2007
Tail of the Tiger

I'm on day five post-chemo #2. The first three days were really not bad at all. One of the highlights of chemo day was being Flocked. For the uninitiated, this means that our lawn was decorated with about 20 plastic pink and red flamingos. They were facing every direction, wings spinning in the wind, looking cheerful and like the zany treat that they were. The day after treatment, the girls and I did a trip to the mall for a few hours, successfully picking out clothing, food and shoes to take us into the fall. The next day, I swam a half hour of laps.

And then comes the time when I'm trying to balance not feeling spaced out with not feeling too nauseous. Plus the fatigue. It's a tricky thing.

I haven't yet sussed out the correct balance of which meds will take care of this. I'm working on it, trying to stay level, trying to catch the tail of the tiger as it swishes by. I just have so much less energy, and that makes me crazy. Maybe tomorrow I'll go for one of the steroidal drugs to carry me through the day.

All this needs to be balanced with my digestive system, which is revolting against all the commotion and disruption to its natural rhythm. I know it'll get better. I just have to wait it out a few more days.

Bad news for Duke and Gale: the kind of anemia I have has nothing to do with iron, so all the red meat won't help. My levels bounced back up, but not quite to pre-chemo levels. The red cell count will probably keep dropping a bit lower until chemo is finished and they can resume their natural cruising speed.

I also got a call back from Driscoll (Plastic Guy). He spoke with my general surgeon (Resciniti) and radiation oncologist (Scholenthaler, the Laser Lady), and they agreed that they could do a tissue expander (to be replaced by an implant) should I choose to go that way. I will still speak with my radiation gal, because I still want to understand her concerns, but I appreciate that the plastic surgeon took the time to connect with them. He also expressed interest in what I will learn from the woman doing the external prostheses. The ongoing amassing of information continues.

I've figured out that my wig makes me feel like I could walk onto the set of Hairspray. It really isn't bad, it just isn't quite what you'd normally expect from my head of hair. I'll wear it to work tomorrow, see how it goes. I've been calling it The Critter, which is not to degrade it; I just can't stop the image of Bobcat, our 23 pound Maine Coon, wearing The Critter.

I had a really difficult moment with my sister. I had sent her pictures of my new look because other people seeing them had reacted so positively. What I could not anticipate was that it would instead be upsetting for her. She felt that I was being insensitive in sending them to her because they were a reminder that I am sick. In fact, I sent them because I *don't* look sick, and that is what people have said. My good intentions had exactly the reverse effect. This made for some difficult conversations until we figured out what had happened. It threw me off center that I could be so off the mark, and made me worry that I was affecting other people this way, too. Duke, Gale, and Kate reassured me that this was not the case. I hope they're right.

September 5, 2007
I'm not going

I've decided that I don't like this chemotherapy stuff, and I'm not going to do it anymore. (I wish.) I have moved out of the three-toed sloth imitation phase into something closer to the Queen of Quease.

It's always exciting to see what might hold some appeal in the eating department. As I was putting together a tuna sandwich for Gale's lunch, the cat and dog were in attendance. The cat jumped up to slurp the liquid being squeezed from the can, and the dog awaited his turn to lick the can itself. With their eager interest, it seemed like something I ought to try. And so, after making Gale's sandwich, I opened another can, and ate tuna fish at 7 a.m. With mayo and relish, of course. Mmmmm. A couple of hours later I went for a waffle, a more traditional breakfast food.

At least today I'm not quite so spacey. All my experimentation with the meds this time has not produced a major reduction in the quease, but we'll see. I seem to feel better later in the day, and what is on the docket for later in the day today?

A boat ride, of course.

This one is with Duke's work. It's a gorgeous day, and I can think of nothing more appealing than cruising into Boston harbor as the sun goes down on the water, but I'm not sure if my presence is fair to everyone else, or myself.

It grates on me that something that would normally be fun is something that I have to think hard about and possibly decide against just because of a little unsteadiness on my pins. I could even bring a scarf to make sure that the Critter doesn't decide to head overboard, or attach a little elastic around the bottom. Wouldn't that be fetching? I could take it off and wave to people on shore, or let other people try it on. So many options.

This whole experience brings new meaning to "wait and see". Things change so quickly; it takes a moment-by-moment assessment of what is possible. Stay tuned.

September 6, 2007
Cure for the Quease

One boat ride, followed by a lobster dinner, followed by a boat ride in the dark, with the lights of the cities and islands around. All in perfect calm 70-degree weather, with your honey and friends.

September 9, 2007
Wig Adventures

I went to the bank yesterday.

Even at 10:30 in the morning, it was already 7,000 humid degrees, and after spending 45 minutes at the town fair, I was a bit depleted. I entered the air-conditioned bank, and spotted one open teller.

As I approached, she spoke up. "Oh, it's you! Hi, Mrs. Stafford! Your hair! It's different! It looks great!"

I was caught a little off guard. Although I have certainly been to this teller before, we have never exchanged more than the typical pleasantries.

"Oh...thank you!" I managed.

"What? Don't you like it?" she asked me immediately.

"Oh, yes. I do like it!" I replied. I smiled, considered telling her a little more about it, because I really don't mind if people know. I glanced around and realized that everyone in the bank was now looking our way.

With the new open structure of the bank (which I like so much) and the teller's enthusiastic greeting, everyone was drawn to our conversation. Would this be the time to remove the wig, wave it at everyone, and declare, "Hey, just been doing a little chemo, guys! Feeling great, though!"?

I paused, elected not to address them all. We told each other to have a nice weekend, and I strolled out with the wig in place and a smile on my face.

I have chosen this wig because I think it is the one that most resembles my hair as it was. I'm thinking, seamless transition here. It is similar in color, is curly, but is definitely more of a just-out-of the-beauty parlor look than I typically manage.

There were a few clients I saw this week who for one reason or another I had not seen for several weeks. They were, therefore, unaware of my New Hair status, and as I expected, they noticed and commented immediately. I used this as an entrée to tell them a bit about what was happening with my Breasty Business.

They are uniformly supportive and well-wishing. But in terms of my hair (which after all, is the topic del día), I had anticipated some reaction from them, and was ready to address it in the comforting privacy of my office. I have been ill-prepared for a public acknowledgement of my new coif.

You would think that I might possibly learn from this experience and be prepared for the next public appearance of the 'do. Piffle.

We went out to my friend Susan's birthday party last night. I'd been looking forward to it, and I was pleased that the timing of it was such that I felt great, with lots of energy for dancing and celebrating. And of course, there would be people there who we've known for years.

We were in the door two minutes, having greeted the birthday girl and her husband, and the next person we saw was Dickie, who I've known longer than most of the others; he was the best man at Susan and George's wedding 23 years ago, and I was the maid of honor.

"Hey, Meg! How are you? New hair! It looks great!"

"Hey, thanks! You, too, can have hair like this," I told him.

A confused look crossed his face. "Really?" he asked.

"Absolutely!" I assured him.

I was about to launch into the briefest of explanations; I've known Dickie for years and felt comfortable letting him know what's going on. At that moment, more guests arrived, and we were interrupted by happy partygoers.

I refrained from just popping off my wig and placing it on his less-than-full head of hair; this party was not about me, after all. The moment passed, and I contented myself with allowing Dickie to remain uninformed. If the opportunity presented itself later in the evening, I could talk to him then. If not, it would fold into the evening of conversation unnoticed by anyone as anything out of the ordinary.

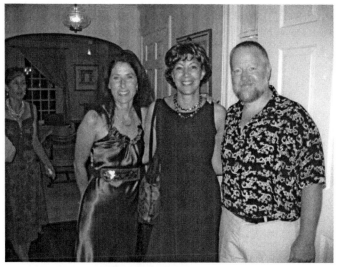

With birthday girl Susan and Duke

I have learned that I have choices about what I say to people and when. I don't know how long my restraint will hold regarding surprising people with an abrupt wig removal, or whether my own imagination around it will be enough. Time will tell.

On a more serious note, my appointments this week have netted the following information:

1) Dolly is no longer in need of draining, having officially abandoned her competition aspirations. Next visit to the surgeon is not for two months.

2) Laser Lady is fine with radiating with the tissue expander in place. She wasn't worried about efficacy, but did have two concerns.

   One was not wanting to delay radiation until the expander was fully expanded, which usually happens over a period of months to gradually stretch the skin. My plastic surgeon wants to put it in place already expanded, and has spoken with my general surgeon about the viability of doing this. She agrees that there would be enough skin to accomplish this.

   Her second concern was about potential complications from surgery. If someone comes to her with the tissue expander in place (but not fully expanded), and then wants to radiate, there are concerns about the skin tightening, causing both pain to the patient and possible contracture, which could require another surgery to correct. By planning with other care providers, these concerns are reduced.

3) At my Ralph (Nadir) visit with Dr. Hugs, I learned that I am on track with my numbers and blood counts. We talked about the difference between the first and second treatments, and what we might be able to do to reduce the nausea/spaceyness on days four, five, and six. He's going to think about it, and we'll talk about it at my next treatment on the 19th.

I have an appointment next week to meet with the woman who now has insurance-reimbursed external prostheses that are custom molded to a woman's body and adhered directly to the skin. All my other care providers are interested in this, as it is relatively new.

September 12, 2007
Symptom Du Jour

I was lulled into complacency once again by feeling well and getting past day 10 without major mouthy issues (the literal ones). But there, lurking under my desk, or behind my file cabinet, was the next surprise, waiting to ambush me.

It was a cold sore that leaped onto my lip right in the middle of a meeting with a client. I could feel it blossom, expanding my lip; it was not until I had the opportunity to consult a mirror that I realized it had the appearance and charm of an earthworm on my face. My family assures me that they had to look carefully to see that it was swollen and red, and I'm trying to buy it.

I called the nurse to make sure that I had the right medicine.

"Oh, no," she declared. "That stuff will take care of any issues inside your mouth, but if you can see it, you need something topical. I'll call in a prescription."

Good thing we're already discussing that house addition for my meds, because the arsenal is being fortified. She promised to call it in before end of day.

For some reason this brought me down. It's not a big deal, it's not permanent, and it's not that painful, but it bummed me out. I just didn't have the energy for something that I hadn't anticipated.

Another medication. Another issue. DAMN IT.

Fortunately, it was a beautiful day, and I was getting ready for a bike ride. This helped as it always does, salve for what ails me. I biked to the Stow airport, which is about eight miles away. Not a pressured ride, but long enough to tucker me out. I went to pick up the prescription, but she evidently forgot to call it in, so I bought something over the counter, and we'll see how that works.

I also had my visit with the lady who does the external prostheses. The woman who had her appointment before me was a number of years older, and when she came out she looked a little shaky. As they opened the door, I heard Mary (the owner) say something about her surgery date, and when to call her. For this woman, the issue was immediate. I'm sure I'll feel differently when I am closer to my own date.

Actually, Mary calls her prostheses non-surgical breast reconstruction.

She makes a mold of the woman's entire chest, and sends this off to a place in Georgia where it takes 8 weeks to be made. They take a symmetrical image of the other breast, then make a mold of the chest wall, and use 21 skin shades to create the prosthesis.

She doesn't even do the fitting until several months after surgery. She waits until all treatment is done, because the body can continue to change, and she wants to wait until it is settled out and weight-stabilized. She says that there is also an emotional component; that a woman needs to be ready and have her expectation level in the right place.

It looks very much like the natural breast, except that (obviously) it isn't. It is not skin, as realistic looking as it is. It sticks to the body with an adhesive that is painted on, and the whole thing is removed at the end of the day. It's waterproof, so you can swim in it and wear it with a regular bra.

This is a terrific alternative, but I need to do some thinking about the whole thing. This is for real. It's a lot to digest, and I need to talk to people, weigh pros and cons. The fact that I feel there is a choice is a good thing. I'm glad that I'm exploring this now, because it is a huge advantage for me to know what to expect, whatever I decide. The clearer the vision of what is to come, the better I can prepare myself.

I realize from questions some of you have asked that I must not have reported that the genetic testing came back negative. I heard a number of weeks ago, but it must not have made it into a missive. So we're talking about a single mastectomy, and no other surgeries (hopefully).

Also, and this is a complete non-sequitur, the wig is doing well. To satisfy some of your curious selves, the cost of synthetic wigs starts around $500. The blend of synthetic and natural is up a few hundred from there, and the all natural ones are up a few to several hundred from there. Insurance covers $350. I chose a synthetic one, but it has a couple of features that bumped up the price, which are that it's very lightweight and also has a lace front, which makes the hairline look more natural. It came in at $700, but I decided that the extra was worth it because it was the one I liked the best, and I have to live with it for a number of months. So all that I might have saved in hair products and haircuts, I spent in one swell foop on the Critter. And my insurance company has already reimbursed me for its half (yea Harvard!).

I had taken it off and was on my way upstairs last night, and I waved at Gale, who was on the phone and working on a project.

"I shake my wig in your general direction," she said. Which was exactly what I was doing.

And I am on my way to bed now, too. Will send more as I filter through my choices. As always, thank you for your kind words and support. I thought about it a lot as I cycled through the hilly green ride, looking at turtles and rabbits along the way.

September 16, 2007
Not so cold or sore

The prescription stuff, which comes in a cute little tube the size of my pinky finger, had a co-pay of 35 bucks. Hot damn.

And the medication did help quickly; it's not completely gone now, but the swelling went down, and it's healing nicely. It was never terribly noticeable anyway, and now I'm armed should it recur.

I had a great time in the kitchen this week. I loved baking cakes for Duke's birthday now that he has joined the ranks of the over 50. I even cooked a whole meal on Friday night. I love to putter in the kitchen, and it was a thrill to feel well and to have the energy, time, and inclination to put the whole thing together, small pleasures expanding. And it's a delight to share them with friends and family.

Every once in a while I catch a glimpse of the temporaryness of all this.

I will not always be watching the quizzical expression on someone's face as she tries to place me, and realize that it is my hair which is confounding her. I will not always be anticipating treatment, planning for the tricky days and the ones when I know I'll feel well. I will not always be taking my hair on and off like a hat, or trying to twirl my hair when I'm driving and realizing, again, that either 1) there is none, or 2) it's synthetic. I will not always be sorting through information, trying to decide about surgery.

There will be some trying, scary times ahead, but they, too, will be temporary. I'll need to remind myself of that during the difficult times.

And this is such a precious year. We are looking at colleges with Gale, and it is Kate's first year at Parker. I do not want to lose any of it; I want it slowed down to a pace that I can savor and relish.

Mostly. It's an intense mix.

Wednesday is the next treatment day, followed by acupuncture on Thursday for the first time. My oncologist concurs that it does seem to help with symptoms from the chemotherapy, although he does not understand why. Can't argue with results, though. Onward!

September 17, 2007
DANG!

Duke keeps telling me to expect the unexpected. And this week's unexpected thing is that chemo did not happen. My counts were too low (can't count on them…) Dr. Hugs keeps assuring me that it was not anything that I did or didn't do, and that it is not an indicator of anything else. They just do not want to put me at any greater risk for infection, so no chemo today. It'll be next Wednesday instead, which, of course throws my entire schedule off; both Ralph visits, *and* my client schedule. Next time, they will give me Neulasta, the drug that helps the immune system bounce back, so on the fourth visit I'll be able to get chemo for sure.

We also talked about the Taxol and agreed that I will do it. This chemotherapy is more user friendly, easier to tolerate, and most people can have it every other week without the Neulasta, so we scheduled the first of those, and will decide whether to do every other, or every third week as we have done.

Grrrrrr. So it goes.

Well, I've got to get started on my bevy of phone calls to rearrange things. At least I was not robbed of my visit with my friend Roe, who kindly drove me to the scheduled appointment.

September 18, 2007
Question

With my next treatment tomorrow, I'm beginning to think about how to ease the quease next week. We have already established that the best thing to do is aim for a boat ride on Day 6. In thinking some more about this, and my practice, I wondered: If Freud had owned a boat, where would he dock it?

And the answer is: in a Freudian slip, of course!

September 23, 2007
Silver Lining

I knew there would be one; I just wasn't sure how soon it would be clear what it was. It actually happened pretty swiftly in this case.

The medical one was that when Susan mentioned to George that I did not get treatment because my counts were too low, he said that was good news. Why? Because it means that we know that the drugs are having an effect on my system. Sometimes people don't experience much in the way of side effects, but they may also not be getting a lot of benefit from the treatment. Some people don't metabolize certain foods; evidently, something similar can happen with heavy metal (all my words, not George's). So, we know that it's getting in there, and my system is responding.

Okay, I'll take that. It's a good spin, and I know that George would not respond this way if he didn't mean it.

Also, I was offered free tickets to North Shore Music Theatre's production of Forever Plaid on Thursday. I would normally be working, or if I had had the treatment on Wednesday, could not have considered this venture for Thursday. But as it was, I had cleared my day entirely, and Gale and I were able to take advantage of this delightful show.

And yesterday I was able to do my first bike ride with my college friend Ana (our typical 20-mile route through Concord and Carlisle) since June. Such beautiful days, these past few. I've been walking (which Charlie, or Mr. Dog as we call him, greatly appreciates), and last night we were out past midnight seeing the touring version of So You Think You Can Dance.

I'm grateful. I had a flash of worry that I would be lulled into forgetting that I was in the midst of a lot of treatment, but no worries. There are plenty of reminders; my port, my hair, my left arm numbness.

When I saw Dr. Hugs and we were talking about planning the next round of chemo, he said that some people with type-A personalities needed to plan that far ahead. Excuse me? Back up. What were the implications here, exactly? Surely I am no more than an A- personality, or perhaps even a B+. Just because I'm trying to get college visits, clients, and fun stuff into my autumn, does that make me Type A?

Not that it's a bad thing; our friend Luc, who spent a year in Taiwan, may have developed a Taipei personality. Anyway, it's another smashing day to enjoy now that we're full of pancakes....

September 26, 2007
Keeping it Fresh

I certainly espouse the notion that it is always good to be trying new things, keeping the marital relationship from becoming stale or routine. With my third treatment today, on our 20th anniversary, I was unexpectedly presented with a unique opportunity for my betrothed and me. The Neulasta arrived as planned yesterday at Emerson, and they were keeping it chilled for me. I had thought that I would receive this as part of today's treatment, but no, it is to be administered between 24 and 48 hours after the treatment, meaning tomorrow. Ish.

The best place to inject is in the fatty part of the upper arm, which makes it difficult to self-administer. I volunteered Duke for this task, and the two nurses who were there just stared at me, with similar looks of something between skepticism and confusion on their faces.

Both said nothing for a moment.

"He'll be okay with it," I offered confidently.

"He's not here for us to explain to him how to do it," one of them said.

"Well, you teach me, and I'll teach him." More blank looks.

I didn't know what the hesitation was. Did they not believe me? Which part was the confounder?

"What about a neighbor?" one asked.

None of our immediate neighbors know what's going on. I could see this approach. "Hey, by the way, I'm having treatments for breast cancer, and what do you think about giving me a little shot in the arm? I'll show you my hats, and wig, and we can have tea!" If I thought I was getting odd looks from these nurses, I can only imagine what that would bring.

The nurses also offered that I could come back before 5:30 and any one of them would do it. But that would mean another trip back. And I was so sure that Duke would be up for the task.

They did agree, and showed me the already-loaded syringe. The only thing to make sure of is that the needle is actually in before pressing the medicine. Ejecting the medicine into the air would be considerably less effective, to say nothing of the expense. So we have that to look forward to tomorrow evening when I get home from seeing the three or four clients who were too tricky to reschedule. Our first new adventure in the 21st year. I count my lucky stars that I did not even hesitate to volunteer my buddy for this.

This morning Kate asked me to fill a tiny bottle with conditioner to take with her to Becket, her 3-day school trip. She handed me the enormous bottle and the teeny one with a minute opening. I started filling the dense liquid into the tiny hole.

"Kate," I pointed out, "I'm going to have hair again by the time I get this thing filled!"

"Hey, good one," Gale called from the other room.

"Have fun at Becket," I called as they were heading out to the car.

"Thanks. Have fun at chemotherapy!" Kate replied.

Yep, it's all becoming just that normal.

Chemo did go fine; my counts were just where they should be. I came home, ate lunch, and went for my second acupuncture treatment. I feel much less spacey than after the last two treatments, and I think more energetic, too. Eating was also key.

Hey, thanks for listening and boosting me through this odd territory.

September 27, 2007
A Shot in the Arm

As I expected, it was pretty much a non-event. We prepared the arm with the alcohol rub, Duke washed his hands, we made sure the syringe didn't have air in it, and he injected. Really not a big deal. I wouldn't exactly recommend it for an amorous evening, but it was not an evening killer either. Took about a minute and we were back to our respective businesses of getting the remote control helicopter to work (Duke's B'day present) and tending to e-mail (guess who).

I had a great day. So good, in fact, that I had a flash of concern that there was only a saline solution in the bag that dripped into me for an hour and a half. There was a handwritten sign that read Cytocin, but I feel so normal today that it makes me suspicious. I'm learning not to look gift horses in the mouth (you never know what they're storing in there).

The two differences this time were the acupuncture treatments and the fact that I skipped the Ativan last night. Not sure which is making the bigger difference, but it doesn't matter. The triumvirate of nausea, fatigue and spaceyness were all at bay today (probably searching out that boat ride that should come on day six). I know enough to know that this does not mean it will be like this every day, but I'm taking each day for what it is.

I started with an hour long walk with my friend Martha and Mr. Dog, and I'm happy to say that it was Mr. Dog who was panting on the way back. Downhill even.

And I put in a few hours at work. Four hours is a great way to go at work.

All this considered together does mean that my sloth imitation may need some work. I have the whole weekend to work on it, including tomorrow, so I better get out my book and start practicing draping myself on the sofa or reclining chair.

My practice suffered its first casualty today in relation to the Breasty Business. One client realized that she was reluctant to call because she felt that her concerns were so trivial compared to what I was dealing with (she didn't find out until earlier this month because of vacations, etc.).

We were able to talk about it today when she came in. She thanked me for all the work we had done together this past year, and told me that I was instrumental in getting her to listen to herself and do what's best for her. In this case, it meant going back to her previous therapist of many years. So perhaps it truly is just another example of doing what's best for her, or at least trying it out. It was important that she not be worrying about me or feeling like she needed to take care of me. Seeing me today made her realize that she didn't have to, that I'm really fine, but this will be an important issue for her to look at in any case.

Other reactions have included concern, elicited cards, flowers, a journal and some ginger, feelings of protection. It's been amazing to see what will come up. This was the first person for whom it was too difficult to stay in treatment, even treatment that had gone well.

Needles to say (that's a pun, not a typo), I'm wondering if the Decadron of this morning is making me chatty, but I'm signing off in any event.

October 1, 2007
The Right Stuff

Any concern that it was not the right stuff has been allayed. I have been working on my sloth thing this weekend, even taking a nap on Sunday, which proves that something other than my norm has been happening. Duke was relieved to know that the shot in the arm was not for naught, and that this stuff is working its way through my system to flush out the alien cells.

I'm glad that I pushed out my work start time to ten o'clock this morning. Would have been a stretch to get in there for eight. We'll see how the day goes. I'm understanding the appeal of coffee, too, which typically serves to wind me up into a large-scale (albeit bald) energizer bunny. Now it seems to bring me up to cruising speed. I have still been able to appreciate the spectacular days, even if I am not out there pedaling away the miles this week. Maybe on the weekend.

October 5, 2007
Fire up the Barbie

No, not the one in pink pumps, Silly. The one that brings back MEAT to the anemic. I started my day with coffee and a sausage (chicken apple), and had salad with Ana for lunch (I ate the bacon from both).

Then I found out at today's Ralph visit that my red blood count is low. If it gets much lower, they pile on Procrit or something else to give it a boost. And my red blood count had been holding steady after that first dip, until now. So whoever told me that eating meat doesn't matter is probably wrong, because when I was making a more concerted effort to eat it, my counts were up. At the very least, it can't hurt, so bring on the steaks!!!

My white blood cell count had spiked as a result of the Neulasta. Yea!! And the nurse said that if I were going to experience bone pain as a result, it would have already happened. And I didn't. So I'm going to give that particular side effect a miss. How cool is that?

I asked if the bump in white blood cell count would head off some of the other mouthy side effects. She said that they were just teeny tiny white blood cells, and probably wouldn't make a difference. And how long do they take to mature? I asked. "About two days," was the answer. So doesn't that support my theory that with the plethora of them now in attendance, some of them could possibly spend some time in my mouth making sure I don't need the rinse and spit?

Personally, I thought that a cold sore was trying to pop its way through yesterday, and I told it not to give me any lip, and so it hurried back where I couldn't feel it. Smart. Anyway, I've expended whatever energy was lurking, and it's time to get to my meeting. Hope the following is coherent.

October 7, 2007
Acupuncture

Yesterday I had my fourth acupuncture treatment in total, and my second with the new person. I am still taking in how different the experience was with each of the two providers. I have every confidence that both are competent, knowledgeable and experienced; it is the difference in each of their approaches that I found so remarkable.

My unsettledness with the first experience revolved at least in part around the fact that I had to keep prompting her to get information about what she was doing.

We talked for a few minutes, and then she said, "I'm going to give you a treatment."

I hopped up on the table, and without further ado, she started inserting the tiny needles into various points (after feeling my pulse and abdomen).

"What are you doing?" I asked.

It was at this point that she started to explain a bit about the meridians, and which ones she was trying to affect. The kidney and liver (metaphorically, not literally) carry a lot of the energy that needed shifting. She inserted the needles into my feet, wrist, abdomen, and three into each ear.

We chatted and discovered that she had done the Pan Mass the same year as I did, and no other years. (The Pan Mass is a 2-day, 200-mile bike ride to benefit the Jimmy Fund. My riding pal, Ana, and I had signed up only for Day 1, 85 miles.) The next year she (Acupuncture woman) went on to do a 450-mile ride through the Rockies. (Whoa! How long did it take to train for that?!) When she was finished, she pulled a light blanket over me, told me that she would leave me for 15 minutes, and that I should try to rest. I did indeed rest, and I'm pretty sure I caught some shut-eye before she returned. I don't recall experiencing a lot around the needles themselves.

After she was back in the room, she was behind me while I lay on the table, and I caught a whiff of something burning.

"What am I smelling?" I inquired.

"Oh, that's an herb, moxa, which is used in conjunction with the acupuncture. It looks kind of like a cigar, and I will use it to warm up the needles. She showed me, and then held it near the groups of needles before removing them. She suggested I return weekly, and in particular to try to get back before my next chemo treatment.

I did schedule some appointments, although I felt a bit uneasy. I realized that although we had connected around the biking, I felt odd that I had to keep prompting her for information when this was my first time experiencing acupuncture. There was something about her manner that was not a good match for me. She was certainly not rude in any way; I am just someone who does better knowing what's going on.

Now, having had two experiences with Ted, the second acupuncturist, I am amazed at the difference in approach. I felt included in every step with Ted. He gathered more particular information and did a couple of different types of treatment. He paid attention to my tongue as a source of information, and also treated my shoulders, which typically hold tension. Rather than feeling like I had a treatment done to me, I felt that I was part of the treatment.

He taught me some Qi Gong as well, something that I can do myself at home to enhance the treatment. It is a moving meditation, which again is a good match for me, as I need to move. We met twice in a row, and will meet again next week, and then he will evaluate when the next time should be. It isn't a prescribed thing. It's individual and personal.

I feel that he paid particular attention and that he does this with each patient or client. I feel I am learning, which is exciting. There were times when he inserted a needle that I felt an electric current emanate from that spot. The energy is literally discharging. Other times there was a tingling, sometimes a little jolt or ache that lasted less than a second. He took time to find those particular points, using pressure on my ankles, for instance, to find the imbalance. Where there was very slight sensitivity, there was receptivity for the needle to help shift energy.

As I am a complete novice, I may well be using terminology incorrectly or inaccurately. I am intrigued to learn more, and to see how it will affect my experience as we go along.

October 11, 2007
We'll Meat Again

So I realized that I have not mentioned how terrific this last week has been. Friday, as I mentioned, I started the day with sausage and coffee. Then Not Your Average Jew's for lunch (certainly Ana, a Catholic school raised gal, and I qualify as not your average Jews), and then once I found out about my red blood cell dip, I had a hot dog as a snack. (For those of you who are not from the Boston area, the real name of the restaurant is *Not Your Average Joe's*. I am compelled to play with this name early and often.) My energy level bounced back quickly, and on

Saturday, Duke and I did a 16-mile bike loop to Stow. Awesome!

The next night, there were no less than three types of red meat at our joint dinner: buffalo burgers (Trader Joe), Omaha burgers (Gail), and steak tips (Stockwells)!! It was a veritable smorgasbeef! And each one so tasty, too!

The next night we were treated to steak, courtesy of our friends Jane and Roger. There is no need for me to ask where's the beef: I know now. I have felt great all week. I realized that it really took until last Friday for my nausea to completely go away, but once it goes, it goes.

I also spoke with my DIEP contact about her surgery. She was incredibly gracious. There's nothing like calling up a complete stranger and asking "Hey, how do you like your breasts?" This was a good choice for her, and it was helpful to hear about the sequence of it; how long the surgery was, how long after all her treatment it occurred (almost a year after the initial lumpectomy), and what the issues are/were. I will talk to her surgeon.

Looking at the last round of AC next Wednesday. Probably my halfway mark for chemo.

By the way, I have been wearing my critter pretty much all the time when I'm out of the house. It's as easy as a hat. One of the perils of wearing it at home, though, is that when I cook, I have to stay out of the way of steam or heat! Both of these things can permanently uncurl any of the curls, and just affect the wig badly. It's hard to remember not to take things out of the oven, or not to take spaghetti out of boiling water! Got to enlist the fam for these tasks, or just put my wig to the side, which is another good option. Yesterday I did this, setting it on top of a lamp in the hallway. Also, I found one of Kate's thin sports head-bands to put on my own fuzzy do. All it needed was a tiny bow on it, and I would look just like a one-year-old (kind of…).

October 14, 2007
Zenith

If 10 days after a treatment is the Nadir, then the weekend before my treatment must be the Zenith, especially when there's a magnificent weekend like this one, full of crisp air and blue skies. I had a great walk with Mr. Dog, who is now starting to request them, and a bike ride out to the Stow airport and back, plus a fabulous anniversary dinner at No. 9 Park. Kate's soccer team trounced their opponent, and Gale interviewed at Wesleyan.

And if Gale didn't have enough of Dolly at home, she traveled today to NYC to see the Dalai's llama at the behest of her friend Si. And where is the Dalai convening the masses? Where is he strutting his stuff? Why at Radio City Music Hall, of course.

Please forgive me if I am irreverand (irreverent??), but we spent part of last night trying to picture this. Do you suppose he is out in front of the Rockettes, or perhaps flanked by them? And what is he wearing? Will this be Dalai the musical? Will he kick up a fuss? The incongruity of these two entities intrigues me, and makes me think that he must have a sense of humor. People of his stature usually do. I am keenly interested to hear about this experience.

The other thing that has been striking this weekend is my awareness of how the ripples of my situation flow out. I have seen or been in contact with people who are just finding out. The classmates and colleagues I saw at an executive coaching conference—except for the ones I have been in regular contact with—were unaware of my situation. When I see people in person, my hair is a great lead-in to conversation, because people comment.

I also received cards from two different people who I have not seen or been in contact with for over 10 years! One heard by running into a mutual friend, and the other heard from her mother, who is friends with my mother. I've also sent e-mails to dear friends who are far away, and with whom I have not been in regular contact. People are uniformly warm, supportive, and loving, which is not surprising for who they are, but still incredibly moving and humbling.

When I run into people, I can always tell when someone knows by the way they respond to me. There is something special in the way they ask how I am, a particular focus in listening to my response. Or they may tell me directly that they have heard. Either way, although it sometimes catches me off guard, I am struck by the natural way that news travels, by people's curiosity and interest.

I am unaccustomed to being the object of news. I try not to call attention to myself; I am living my life, I don't want to be the focus of attention. Yet at the same time, I am appreciative of everything that people have to offer. I am in the unique position of receiving help when I least expect it, and of sometimes having to ask for help when I least expect to need it. It is forcing me to learn a way of interacting that is at once awkward and rewarding. I am humbled and awed by the connection to people, by the willingness of others to be present and available sometimes before I even realize the need myself. This is preparation for the surgery in January, which will be more altering and a bigger challenge than anything I have faced so far.

October 15, 2007
Hooray for Dalaiwood!

Gale reports that there were many lamas there. Have you already herd? They wore New Balance (of course) sneakers with their robes. I was disappointed to hear that they did not do a single group number (probably trying not to compete with Spamalot). But I understand that the Dalai Lama himself was impressive, and talked about Peace and Prosperity, and that he does, indeed, have a good sense of humor.

October 19, 2007
Sloth Weekend

I completed my last round of Adriamycin and Cytocin on Wednesday.

Yea! Felt okay yesterday and did go into work for a few hours. I'm hoping my meds kick in soon today. Both nights' sleep were disturbed, the first one by the cats who were demanding sequentially, and then when I finally had them squared away I was called by the Littleton public schools (which neither of my children attend) at 6 a.m. to tell me that school would be delayed because of a water main break. Last night the earthquake woke me up, and both times I had trouble returning to sleep, which I attribute to the meds (blame it all on the meds).

Because of the recent publications about Taxol, Dr. Hugs is again questioning the usefulness of my taking this drug. We already know that it is not of huge benefit for someone with my profile, so the question really is whether it is of any benefit. We're talking small percentages here, but the other side is, why not do it? I have tolerated the first round of chemo well, which is usually the most difficult one to bear. For the Taxol, they do not give nearly the amount of ammunition in terms of anti-nausea meds, and people usually do not need Neulasta in order to be infused with Taxol every two weeks instead of every three. However, as with any type of chemotherapy, response to treatment is highly individual, and some people do get sick on Taxol. We will revisit this next Friday at my Ralph appointment.

In the meantime, I have an appointment scheduled for Dec. 14 (soonest available) with *the* guy at Beth Israel Hospital who does the DIEP flap procedure. I felt I owed it to myself to at least talk to him.

And now I'm coming into Sloth weekend. Just for the record, I have an affection for these furry, benign creatures; I actually did a little paper on them in sixth grade. I am astounded at their capacity for inactivity while still remaining viable as a species. It is in no way derogatory when I refer to them. It is just that their proclivity for relaxation is something that I am not always able to achieve.

However, on a weekend following heavy-duty drugs, I am able to get there much more easily. I usually require fairly rigorous exercise in order to chill properly. In many ways, it is nice to have my Paretsky novel be one of my main priorities. It's just hard to give up the things I expect to be doing. I do like to putter, but I can't plan much, so I look for movies to watch, etc. If it's raining, so much the better; all the easier to hang out and relax.

October 20, 2007
Earthquake!

There have been a couple of questions about the earthquake I referenced. Evidently, we Littletonians had our own personal earthquake the other night. It jolted Duke and me out of bed, but the girls' sleep remained undisturbed.

Earlier in the day, Bobcat had fallen out of the window when only Kate was home. She heard a crash, but could not see any damage, and realized that she could not find the cat, either. After searching the house twice (with the aid of the dog and the other cat), she finally heard him meowing on the front porch, demanding to be let in. Duke arrived home a half hour later, and realized that the cat had inadvertently pushed out the screen next to his window bed. Yes, his 23-pound girth must have shoved just a tad too hard. Thankfully, his (Bobcat's) bed is next to a first floor window, making the fall only about ten feet. He appears undamaged and unrattled as far as we can tell. But it meant that our first concern when we heard the noise was to go running downstairs in search of the cat.

He, too, was up and looking around, as was Daphne, our other cat. But all is well, and our 2.5-on-the-Richter-scale earthquake seems to have done no other damage than disturbing our sleep. Weird.

One foliage note: with all the rain we had last night, the trees have all turned into a burst of yellow, finally! It's sunny without being sunny!

On a completely different note, Kate is getting to know some of her classmates. She was in a class and two girls sneezed.

"I can't get sick," one girl said.

"Me either," Kate replied.

"No, I really can't get sick," the girl insisted.

"Me either," Kate responded.

"No, you don't understand," the girl explained. "My mother's going through chemotherapy."

"Mine, too!" Kate replied. The girls talked, learned that it was different illnesses, and types of chemo, but still such an odd way to forge a friendship. It is a bittersweet moment for me to hear about. I want her to connect with people, but like this?

Numb and Number

Okay, so the fatigue is not as bad as I thought, at least so far, but it is the quease and the achiness that is getting me. The achy part is newish. I've had a little bit in the past in my shoulder blades, but now my entire back, rib cage, chest and neck are tender to the touch. This may be the Neulasta talking, although it seems a little early. Tylenol does seem to be helping, but this robs me of one of my greatest comforts, which is back rubs and just plain hugs. Well, the hugs just need to be gentle. The whole thing has me just a tad peeved and grateful that this is the last of this round of nastiness.

I am prepared to go ahead with the Taxol, because with the unknown benefit, or even small benefit, now is the time to do it. If I experience bad side effects, like neuropathy in my limbs, I'll stop. I have no desire to pollute my system with something unnecessary, but I do not want to avoid a potential benefit. Hugs (the doctor variety) will be agreeable. We'll just need to negotiate the interval between treatments, but that shouldn't be an issue either. I will take the holidays into account, and my reaction to the first dose (which I can't even imagine right now). In the meantime, I am looking to dump the quease. Sleazy queasy.

So what's with the numb and number? Well, numb would be my left arm. Number would be, oh, zero for more treatments, or many for the amount of apples it will take to make one gallon of cider at the apple press event this afternoon. Or four for the number of pumpkins we will need to carve next weekend. Or 67 for the number of sips of ginger ale I need to take to get through a bottle. Or one for the number of large screen TVs that arrived at our house yesterday. Or three for the number of days until I can vanquish the quease (probably). Or one for the number of minutes until I head for a new book.

I did, in fact, nap through the second quarter of the Pats game. But I woke up, and Duke and I took Mr. Dog for a long walk in the beautiful Indian summer day. The soreness seems to have extended into my limbs somewhat. I had not previously been able to achieve this level of soreness without a major tumble on a ski slope. It's very weird, and (damnit) better be short-lived. I looked wistfully at the bikers going past, and am just glad that I could get out there at all before the leaves depart completely.

October 23, 2007
Sore No More

The soreness mostly left by Monday morning. I was fighting the quease all day, which meant that I was pretty beat by the end of a 7-hour work day. I couldn't summon the energy to attend my coaching group, which means that I was really tired.

By the end of today, I started to feel better all around, which allowed me to discover a fun new game called Quease Shop (not a Monty Python skit). Actually, it's probably better named End of Quease Shop. I'm not all the way there, but going through the Hannaford Supermarket in Ayer meant that everything looked inviting (OOOOH LOOK! COTTAGE CHEESE!!! How exciting!).

And then...chocolate cluster-flavored Life cereal! Mmmmmm... organic salsa with roasted corn. Wow. It's all so fascinating and appealing. Guava-flavored soda! Why not? I'm thrilled with all of it! How many of these things could I combine and eat on the way home? Which ones might not show if dribbled down my shirt? Salad (with ham) still wins the day in the end, but our cupboards now boast the creativity of those colorful aisles, and the girls are happy with the booty.

It feels good to be surfacing from these days when I don't even realize how hard I'm working just to stay level. It may rain tomorrow, but I know it will feel good just to be outside, or smelling the coffee brewing, or snapping my fingers to Roy Haines.

October 24, 2006
Chemo Brain

This is a term I heard recently that refers, I think, to difficulty remembering or organizing things. While I have not seemed to suffer from this too much, it does provide a most excellent explanation for the following. Ginger, by the way, is known for its nausea reducing qualities, so I have been experimenting with it in various forms.

Quease Shop
A MAN walks into a shop and approaches a GENTLEMAN behind the counter who is wearing a tuxedo.

Man: Have you got any ginger ale?
Gentleman: No.
Man: Well, then have you got any ginger snaps?
Gentleman: No, sorry, we haven't.
Man: Well, then how about some fresh ginger? Or pickled?

Gentleman: No, and no.

Man: What about ginger tea? Gingerbread? Carrot ginger soup?

Gentleman: No. Wait a minute…no, and no.

Man: Ginger beer at least?

Gentleman: No, absolutely not.

Man: Well then, what have you got? This is, after all, a quease shop!

Gentleman: We've got oats.

Man: OATS? Why have you got oats?

Gentleman: Because this is a shop of OAT QUEASINE!

October 28, 2007
Nadir #4

I know when I'm starting to compose an e-mail in my head that it's time to get it down on paper (virtual paper, anyway). It takes up too much room in there, so if I download it, it keeps the memory storage intact (kind of).

I had my Nadir visit and Nadir Moment on Friday. I had a great morning, going into Boston to meet with my coaching client, then stopping at an Open Studio craft fair on my way back, before proceeding to Emerson for my visit. I could feel my energy wane, but I was in a good mood. I've come to realize that along with my Nadir pattern of anemia, not only do I feel tired, but I have less tolerance generally, and it doesn't take much to make me feel annoyed.

Usually when I arrive for my appointment, the nurse takes me almost immediately to have my vitals checked and to draw blood so they will have my numbers by the time I see a clinician. This time, it was almost 25 minutes before any of the nurses even took me to do this. Next, I was showed to a room to wait for the nurse practitioner. It was another 25 minutes before she appeared.

"Sorry," she said, indicating her quite pregnant belly, "It takes me a while to get down the hall."

Had she apologized for the wait, I would have been fine, but somehow using her pregnancy as an excuse for the lateness rubbed me the wrong way. I was a little impatient and eager to get out of there.

We did need to talk about the Taxol, and What Next in my treatment, except that I would have to repeat this conversation with Hugs because it was a major decision. I told her that I had decided to go through with the Taxol because even with the small potential return, I couldn't leave this stone unturned. She heard me, and supported the importance of paying attention to that in determining a treatment plan.

Then we moved on to what to expect. I knew that the Taxol is generally better tolerated than the Adriamycin/Cytocin cocktail, but she began to explain about the pre-treatment drugs; people often have an allergic reaction to Taxol, so they give steroids in advance, as well as on the day of treatment, in addition to Benadryl on the day of treatment. It means five times the dose of Decadron than I had taken on a day after the other treatment, and it has to be taken 12 hours and then 6 hours before treatment, so it will mean waking myself up to take it, and then getting back to sleep somehow; though if I can't, the Benadryl will surely see to that later in the day.

Ick.

I hate the idea of all that stuff, but it is a package deal. You don't get the heavy-duty stuff without the drugs to help you deal with the likely chain of side effects.

Apart from the day of treatment, however, people generally don't feel nearly as tired, or nauseous as with the AC. Often, people feel a bone soreness/achiness the day or two after, but it doesn't last as long. Also, people often feel a tingliness or numbness in the fingertips or toes. If this goes away by the time of treatment, then it won't last. If it stays until the time of the next treatment, there's a 50 percent chance that it will stay permanently.

I am choosing this. Four separate times. I will be loaded with enough steroids and antihistamines to dry out a watermelon, I'll ache and tingle and I will hope that it is doing something helpful in the long term. Am I nuts? I'm going to continue on with this for another three months of my life?

WHAT THE FUCK? That's what I say.

I rode home in my grumpiness and decided that a boost of beef was just the thing for my anemic self, because I had less than an hour before I needed to ride up to Andover for a work/social evening. Duke was later horrified to learn that I microwaved up an Omaha steak burger (and he properly grilled them that evening for himself and Gale). It did actually help bring me around, or maybe I was just low on fuel generally at that point. Either way, I lost a little of my surliness by the time I reached my destination.

Two days later, I'm moving on. Duke and I did our 16-mile bike loop this afternoon, always key for my mental health. It was one of those days when this whole Breasty Business was in my face (an odd place for it). It can sometimes fade into the background, but it obviously must inevitably take center stage upon occasion.

I had a good wiggy moment the other day. A client was leaving my office, and she asked how I was doing.

Then she leaned toward me confidentially and asked, "Have you started to lose your hair?"

I assured her that I had, and pointed to my coif, and said "Wig!" I do take delight in fooling people, silly as it is. I'm still not a complete Cue Ball; I've got a little fuzz. Not as much as say, a newborn chick, but then we all know that I wasn't born yesterday.

So, on we go. I had a moment last weekend, too, when I just wanted this whole fucking thing to be over. I needed to borrow Duke's shoulder to deposit a small storm of tears. But it passes, and the rest of life moves in, presenting its normalness in a way that is reassuring. World Series, soccer games, parent/teacher conferences, work, picking pumpkins, cats, dog, laundry. It's all part of the rhythm of my life. And this week I have the treat of having no medical appointments. No waiting. No new information (hopefully). Just the good stuff. I'll take it.

November 5, 2007
And On We Go....

Hoping this fine fall weather finds you enjoying the leaves, mild days, and cool nights.

We have two new members of the family, by the way. They are of the rodent persuasion, baby rats that Kate and Gale have named Raoul and Tobin (what else?). They're very sweet and engaging, as the cats will surely tell you.

I've been feeling groovy this past week. I had a call last Monday from a Hugs emissary requesting a meeting, so I dutifully (albeit reluctantly) made an appointment for last Friday. However, I called on Thursday to respectfully cancel, as I did not see the need for a full-blown appointment. I had already gone over the Taxol issues with Nurse Mazzola, and had decided to go ahead with the treatment. Unless he had something very late breaking to bring up, I was ready to proceed, and felt that a phone call would suffice. After all, I had been in the week before. I'm going in this week, so why did I need yet another visit in between? I spoke with the same emissary, who spoke with Hugs. He agreed to call me instead of meeting. In fact, he left a message tonight, and I'll probably speak with him tomorrow.

It's a small thing, but I appreciate that I did not end up having a meeting last week. I have two medical-related appointments this week, two next week, and I haven't looked beyond that. I think it's at least one every week. I will do whatever is necessary; I just didn't feel that this one was. It was good to have a week off, and to have input into that decision. I am not a passive recipient here.

I'm feeling a little nervous about the Taxol, just because it's new. I'm sure it will be fine, but until I actually go through it, I can't be sure. So we'll see. I have been biking and walking as much as time will allow, getting out to hear Molly's band, and even doing some cooking! All so fun!

Too tired to write more now, but there have been some thoughts burbling around in there that will probably coalesce into something more coherent later in the week. Enjoy the lovely fall days!

November 7, 2007
New Idea

I wasn't exactly on time taking my Decadron (a preemptive strike to help deal with the Taxol), but I did get the first five in before 10 p.m., and the second five in at 4 a.m. No trouble dropping back to sleep, but I woke up at 5:30 and bounded out of bed feeling like there was something I should be doing.

Perhaps it wasn't the best idea to have some caffeine in my coffee this morning, because I'm now doing my Energizer Bunny thing. It's cold (30 degrees), but maybe I should leash up Señor Dog for a little stroll. Or I could partake of my latest suggestion for the chemo room: exercise DVDs!

I think that instead of handing us blankets and pillows, they should offer track suits, and slip in a Jane Fonda or Richard Simmons DVD. We would have to make special accommodations for the IV lines. Perhaps we'll use them as jump ropes. This would be easier for the folks with IVs near their wrists, a little more of a challenge for those of us with the ports closer to our necks.

If we exercise vigorously enough, maybe some of our wigs will pop off. Those people would get prizes. You know, chemo room favors, little candies or something. Brightly colored hats, maybe?

For the truly creative, there could be IV Line Dancing, like the gymnasts who twirl those streamers.

Of course, this may all change once the Benadryl hits my system. Depends on how much more Decadron I get first: my own personal little drug war. Which will win out, the up, or the down? Will I fall asleep mid-sentence (probably to the delight of my fellow chemo buddies), or request to do laps around the hospital? We'll find out shortly.

PS: I returned Hugs's call yesterday. I dialed a number from memory, and happened to get a back line that Hugs answered himself! He wanted to let me know that what the research is showing is that for my profile, we already knew that the Taxol is not hugely beneficial, but that doing it every three weeks may be of no benefit, whereas doing it every week or two may be of some benefit. So, we'll be bumping up the frequency of this as long as the side effects don't get in the way. Oh boy!

November 7, 2007
Well Treated

My biggest discovery of today is that IV Benadryl trumps IV Decadron, at least temporarily. Minutes after I received the Benadryl, I became woozy and drowsy. I didn't actually fall asleep, but I did rest for a little while. Then I came around, and could read and chat with Roe, who did yeoman's duty being at the hospital from 9:30-2:30. I'm tired now, mostly from having my system up and then down.

I think a good night's sleep will help me out a lot. So far, not much nausea. Much confusion about the timing of my next dose because of Thanksgiving. We'll sort that out next week. More soon.

November 11, 2007
Shop 'Til It Drops

This expression has taken on a new meaning, as Kate and my mom and I did a little clothing shopping yesterday. There was a lovely velour shirt that I had to try on to see whether it really worked or not. The cut was not quite right, but really the trickiest part was that my wig disappeared into my own shirt as I got it out of the way. I can just imagine leaving it behind for the next woman to find as she brings in her own selection of items to try.

November 11, 2007
Second verse, not the same as the first

So is this a kinder, gentler (albeit less impactful) chemo? I suppose so. I did not receive the heavy hitting anti-nausea drugs, just one plus the steroids and Benadryl, as I have already outlined. By the end of the first night, I was pretty wakeful, bouncing around, and not getting into bed early. The next day I worked several hours, and was pulling pumpkin bread out of the oven at 11 p.m., much to Gale's consternation. I seem to continue to have a fair amount of energy, although I'm hitting a lull right now. Where is the sloth? I think I need a hammock.

There does seem to be some low level of quease going on, and a little achy thing. Not terrible, but I'm not totally myself, either. I'm trying to ignore what I can't change and rest if I need it. This is still unprecedented, so I don't know what to expect. I just know that day one is not predictive of other days.

Mr. Magic, my acupuncturist, asked me how it has been to consider death. I can't remember exactly how he brought it up, actually, just that his tone was conversational, as if asking what I thought about the movie I saw last weekend. There I was, being held at needlepoint (what a stitch!) and suddenly launching into a casual discourse about death. I told him that there hasn't been a lot of fear. From the outset, my prognosis has been pitched as extremely positive, from a number of standpoints, and I am listening to this. My tearier moments have come from the kindnesses of others, and this continues to be true. I get annoyed at the incredible inconvenience, even as I am deeply grateful that there is so much to treat and be thankful for.

Also, as I have felt well from the beginning—apart from the evolving side effects of the chemo—I do not feel like I am "sick." I discovered the initial lump after coming back from a 20-mile bike ride. I have been able to carry on with my life mostly as usual.

I do not even like the term cancer survivor. It implies that one has barely made it through. And surely, this is sometimes the case. There are times that I feel the enormity of the ordeal; but again, mostly I am just living my life, trying for the uncomfortable aspects of it to take up as little space as possible. Perhaps it is this peripheral view that makes this whole experience workable right now. As long as I can look squarely at what decisions I need to make, I can afford the luxury of keeping the rest of it at the corner of my vision.

When I do think about death, it is not scary, perhaps in part because it does not feel like my time. I am much more focused on my life, how involved in it I am, and how much I want to do. The transition to death, when it occurs, will be an interesting one, but just not soon. I do get very choked up even considering leaving my family in this way, both for them, and selfishly for myself. I cannot bear it. I simply cannot.

It turns out that Mr. Magic has looked at death perhaps more squarely, as he had a bout with Lyme Disease earlier this year. He was in cardiac intensive care for three days, followed by three more days in the step-down unit. He said that he felt peaceful, but that his own son is 11, the very age he was when his father died, and that he would not ever want his own son to experience this kind of loss.

I live with no regrets, and I suppose it is this same feeling that propels me to welcome any treatment that can offer a continued insurance policy against recurrence of disease.

Well, this has been cheery, eh what? Part of the deal once in a while.

By the way, my eyebrows have decided to do a slow fade. This in-your-face kind of a symptom is a tad bothersome, because I definitely have to spend a little time filling in with a brush. The no-eyebrows look is kind of a freaky one. Before you know it, I'll be doing a full-blown makeup thing. Who knew?

November 17, 2007
Yew for the Jew

Taxol is derived from the yew tree. Have I already mentioned this to yew all? Its leaves are highly toxic, and less than 100 grams of chopped leaves can off any adult who is silly enough to be sitting around chomping yew leaves. However, a substance derived from the yew bark (which in this case is less bad than its bite) was found to be a potent anti-cancer drug. Yews were almost wiped out because of this until a method of synthesizing part of it was created. There is more from the article that Roe sent to me about the yew, but among its highlights is that the yew is considered the Tree of Life across a number of cultures. How lovely that I am sipping from its benefits as it gets to the root of my problem.

And truly, so far, the bite is less than what I experienced with the Adriamycin, Cytocin cocktail. I'm less tired and less queasy for less time, returning to a more typical energy level much more quickly. My digestive system still took a hit, and I found out yesterday at my Ralph visit that my red blood cell count is down again, but the white blood cells were numerous enough to support a flu shot, which I have never had before now. Hopefully, by increasing my beef and spinach intake, I can still avoid the Procrit or Epogen, but at least my treatment won't be delayed.

I am scheduled for this Wednesday morning. Not ideal, given that we are hosting Thanksgiving, but it's one of those things that is out of my control. If last time is any indicator, I'll be pretty much out of commission on Wednesday, but should be much better on Thursday. I'll have to remember not to eat like a pig on Thanksgiving, but otherwise, I am psyched and looking forward to it.

My visit with my sturgeon, I mean surgeon, earlier in the week reminded me that she is blunt like a sledge hammer, but there is no doubt about where she stands. She still recommends mastectomy. After chemo ends, in mid-December, I will need an MRI and mammogram before I see her again (got to keep my visit count up at all costs). This needs to happen before surgery, which I continue to kick and scream about, but which I will ultimately have, probably mid to late January.

Duke and I watched an excellent DVD from Lina Loo that laid out the options for reconstruction, and the advantages and possible complications of each type. They found some incredibly articulate women to talk about their choices, and why each one was right for her. The most important thing seems to be to go into any one of them with clear expectations. This avoids disappointments and dashed hopes. I'm pretty sure that I'll be going with the tissue expander option. Would I make this same choice if I was much younger or much older or was in a different stage with my kids? Maybe. It's hard to assess, although the importance of my stomach muscles would likely be the same. Priorities vary with timing.

So there we go. It's an odd thing to become chummy with the nurses at Emerson, but I'm in there nearly every week, and on the chemo weeks I'm there for hours. I realized yesterday that I had not made an effort to know their names (and they do not sport them on their uniforms). I'm sure part of this is my resistance to embracing this whole deal. It's not like getting to know the people who work at your gym. But they are a friendly lot, and I do like to greet people by their names, not just respond with "Hey!" So I'll get the names down.

Duke commented the other night that he had not seen my head for a while. I have not exchanged slothiness for ostrichness; I have on either my wig or a little hat at night. Part of this is because with the cooler temperatures, I need a little covering. But his observational comment brought tears to my eyes, making me realize that there was something more than practicalities about this. Sometimes I feel vulnerable, exposed with my baldy dome. A lot of the time I don't even think about it. Again, sometimes it is the unexpected things that produce a reaction. Part of the journey.

From Beth:

Yes, I remember looking into the Yew Tree and Taxol as well… amazing what nature provides…and what our bodies can tolerate. How is the numbness in your toes and fingers and joints?

I became quite close to one of my oncologist nurses and was quite shocked when at our last meeting she said goodbye very fondly, and said she hoped to never hear from me again (her way of wishing me health).

I think these folks are totally amazing in their work and realized after her kind "goodbye" that they must have a hard time keeping close to, but detached from, their patients; they witness and feel so much of the pain for breast cancer patients. Years later, I ran into her at a labyrinth event at Dana Farber and we hugged and laughed and felt so happy to see one another…then said goodbye again. People come in and out of our lives, some for a moment, some for length, some for meaning, and some for their facilitation of some other event or moment, helping to move us along our path.

Happy gobble day to you all.
Xo
Beth

November 25, 2007
Post Thanksgiving

I was up and pretty zippy on Thanksgiving, and we had a grand day with our guests from NYC, Cambridge, and Falmouth arriving within minutes of one another. I do love this holiday of Epicurean bounty, especially as Duke does the lion's share of the cooking. I never visit as much as I would like, but I still love having everyone here, eating the food of the earth, and jostling around the table in various combinations of people and mashed vegetables and pies (the pies aren't mashed).

Friday, my energy was still good, up for a walk with Martha, and a party of pot luck leftovers. Then yesterday I took the drive to New York for a mini-reunion with high school friends. On the way back through Connecticut today, I noticed some unusual signs. There was a road sign for a prison with "(Seasonal)" written underneath. I hadn't realized that the law was a seasonal thing, or that prisons are. Perhaps I have been misinterpreting the phrase "Take no prisoners" all these years. It must be referring to the off season when you're not allowed to take them. Who knew?

And just down the road there was a lit sign reminding us to "CLICK IT or ICK IT. IT'S THE LAW." This must mean to buckle your seatbelt, or…spit on it? That would be the only safe way to ick it while driving, as far as I can tell. Connecticut must be way more quirky than I had realized. I'll have to be careful if Gale ends up going to college there. You think you know a state, and then you realize that it's only a state of mind.

As you can tell, the impact of this chemo is much less in terms of the heavy duty side effects. My gut definitely takes a hit, and I have a low level quease/tummy ache for a few days, but it clearly did not get in the way of my Thanksgiving fun, food, and frolic.

No surgery date yet, but we're inching closer to a plan. As much as I kick and scream, it still appears to make sense to my providers that this happen.

November 29, 2007
Oy Veyn

You know you're deep into medical land when someone tells you that you have beautiful veins and you beam with pride. I have to hand it to the gals at Emerson; they have made it seem easy to take blood on my Ralph visits, and yes, one of them told me I have beautiful veins.

I am having to revise my former status as someone who needed her veins coaxed into giving up a few viles, I mean vials, of blood. I no longer break into a sweat when I see them rip open the needle packet; a dubious kind of progress, but what the hell? I'm not yet up to observing the whole process, but then, that isn't my goal, either. Nice to know that she's thinking about me from the inside; I'm not just a pretty arm.

I saw Hugs on Wednesday. My counts have rebounded (and they're trying out for the NBA). We'll see how they are next Wednesday, but he's assuming we'll be able to go ahead. They're willing to treat with lower white counts because the Taxol does not suppress the white blood cells so much. If the white count is borderline, he may have me get a shot of Neulasta to make sure we can go ahead with the last one. So far, I have not experienced the concerning side effects of the numbness in my extremities.

Hugs said that once chemo stops, people usually return to about 80 percent within a few weeks, and then it takes several months for all the counts to return to their pre-chemo state. I'm slightly anemic but stable, so he's not concerned that I'll be dipping further down. We're not concerned about beefing them up; I'm just trying to eat sensibly (in other words, I use a fork and knife and the occasional spoon…)

I asked if the hair returns along with the other 20 percent. Sounds like it's a gradual thing, and that I should not count on the color. I'm very curious about how it will come back, as I know that the texture, amount of curl, and color can be different. And all these things are easily changed should I so choose. Something to think about in the late spring, I guess.

I contacted the plastic surgeon's office about setting up a surgery date, and this seems to have had some effect because I have now heard from my general surgeon's office about seeing her beforehand (also seeing Plastic Guy beforehand so that he remembers me, and connects the boobular photos that he has with the other body parts). I'm seeing them in the middle of January with an eye toward a late January surgery date. So much fun.

December 3, 2007
Snowy Morning Missive: Discovery

Saturday was another intensive day of learning about the ripples of the Breasty Business news (or creating them). It was the morning of the annual bazaar in Littleton, where local organizations and schools sell all kinds of stuff for the holidays. One of the first people I ran into was the mom of a girl Kate has been friendly with, particularly a few years ago. We had become friendly ourselves, sharing a love of music. She was stationed at a booth that was not too busy, and we chatted for a while.

At some point I let her know what was going on with me, and she replied, "I know. I say a prayer every time I pass your house." She lives about a mile up the road, so she would likely pass by daily, at least. She continued, "I've been a silent supporter. I know that you already have support, and people to bring you food, but there are a whole group of us who are aware and supporting you silently."

A lump rose in my throat. Whoa.

"Wow, thanks, Sue."

"I chose to do it that way. It's fine," she said cheerfully.

I continued my wanderings in the brand new middle school gym. There were high school seniors selling jam they had made, and one of them was a girl who Gale has been friendly with.

"Oh, hi, Mrs. Stafford!" she greeted me. "I like your hair!"

"Thanks! It's a wig," is what popped out of my mouth. "Yeah, doing chemo, so, a wig."

We went on to discuss the jams, and I bought peach and raspberry. I hope I have not ruined her for commenting on people's hair ever again. The poor kid sitting next to her looked a little wide-eyed, but said nothing. Oops.

There was a cruel sign letting us know that we were not supposed to eat or drink in the gym; those peanut butter chocolate cookies would have to wait. I meandered on, arriving at another booth manned by one of Gale's former Destination Imagination coaches. He was encouraging me to participate in the Rotary Club.

"We changed our meeting day to Fridays," he added, which actually works better for me. I told him that I was unlikely to take on a new project soon.

"I hear you were a bit under the weather." He is the first person to approach me in this way.

"Yeah, I'm coming to the end of the first phase," I informed him. "Then I've still got surgery next month, and radiation after that, so it will be a little while before I'm freed up."

Marc is a tri-athlete and has encouraged me to participate in the sprint triathlon that he organizes in Littleton. I have been tempted and was considering it for last year, although obviously it did not happen. He mentioned it again for this coming summer.

"Maybe," I replied.

It would be awesome to pull off this half-mile swim, 10-mile bike ride, and 3-mile run in July. And this year I would be at the young end of my age category. Nice. Again, there may have been a little collateral damaging of the people standing nearby, but c'est la vie. I can't protect everyone.

"Come to a meeting anytime. Consider it an open invitation," was his parting salutation.

I am struck again by how much goes on that is completely outside my awareness. This is always true, but I am awed by the power of what is possible, the currents that carry us. I'm sure that it is part of my lesson in all this to let that in.

Later in the day, I learned that I shouldn't assume that others will share the news regarding my illness. Gale related to me that while she was at the bazaar, she had run into some of her friends from Littleton; also, at yet another booth, she saw the mother of one of her friends, and this was a friend who had visited with us not long after my initial diagnosis. We had mentioned the situation to Gale's friend, so Gale thought that she was safe in assuming the friend's mom would know the situation. Not so.

In this case, word had not traveled, even in the same family. It is so individual; not only our relationships with people, but also how other people process information of this type, what their comfort level is in sharing it with others, or with us. Different personalities respond in various ways, some more introverted, some more extroverted. It is not a matter of right or wrong; it is about what works for each person, at that time.

There's a lot to take in. There are pieces of this Breasty Business that I can anticipate, but there are always some that catch me off guard. That's not a bad thing. It keeps me honest and alert. I'm just not always prepared.

December 6, 2007
3 Down, 1 to Go

Since I have not had an allergic reaction to the Taxol, the amount of steroid I was given yesterday was decreased by half. This is largely a good thing, except that it means the IV Benadryl could take hold more strongly, sending me into la-la land more quickly. Wheee! Within minutes, I was looped out.

It also meant that I dozed on and off after that, surfacing to take my dance partner (the IV pole) with me to the restroom. They call us IV Benadryl recipients a cheap date. Oh yes, what could be more romantic than the chemo room? I can't imagine.

I was more tired last night, too, but didn't go to sleep until after 11. Then I was up at four courtesy of Bobcat, who was interested in food and company. Normally I could just drop back off to sleep, but not today. I seem to remember some sleep oddity last time, too. Maybe the steroid lingers longer than the Benadryl. Who knows? Hopefully I'll sleep well tonight. The nausea is very minimal. I can't get interested in coffee (even decaf) in the afternoon; it just doesn't appeal. But that's no big deal. For once water seems just perfect.

So it looks like January 25 is going to be the surgery date. I'm getting calls about pre-op stuff and meetings with both surgeons as well as Hugs, all separately, of course, just to keep my visit quota intact.

My counts were good yesterday, so that I didn't need Neulasta, and do not have to have a Nadir visit next week. I can just come back in two weeks for the final chemo, and hopefully my counts will be okay then, too. It would be a bummer to have it bumped, (would that make it a bumper?) but it would not change the surgery date.

I need to wait until after that to start preparing myself for that next round. I can focus on only so much at a time. Plus there are holiday festivities to consider.

December 9, 2007
Yewlside thoughts

Once again I was lured into the trap of assuming I would learn from history and thereby know the course of my latest chemical adventure. Primarily this is true, but this time I am experiencing a rather yuckoid taste in the mouth (which is not to say I'm down in the mouth, just down about the taste residing there at the moment). It's not so much nausea as needing the taste of things to be sharp and bold or they're not appealing. I've started raiding Kate's supply of fruity candy to help in this department. This hails back to my very first treatment of AC, when I also found this to be helpful. It's weird, and I'm hoping that it will only last for a couple more days.

Also, my head is tender (I know, I've always been soft in the head). Not terrible, but my wiglet was actually bothering me yesterday. I need to turn the shower strength down or the water becomes uncomfortable. So odd. This, too, will hopefully be short-lived. I have experienced some slight passing numbness in two of my toes, but I'm not sure if this is related to the cold or what. It doesn't last, so that's a good thing.

After two nights of waking at 4 a.m., my sleep has returned to normalish, and even though I have awakened at 4, I have been able to go back to sleep for a couple of hours. It hasn't seemed to diminish my energy level much, and Mr. Dog has been pleased to prance around the snowy neighborhood.

I would still say that this round is not as strenuous as the last, but I think I had fooled myself into thinking that I would not notice it at all, and this is simply not the case. There are still a bevy of chemicals that take a while to get through my system, which is the idea here, and they may sometimes pile up on one another. I need to abandon the notion that I can anticipate completely how I will respond. There just cannot be that level of predictability, no matter how much I would like that to be so.

Let's hope the freezing rain thing stays away. Snow is a much better way to go.

December 12, 2007
It Had to Be Yew....

It has taken a little longer this round to return to whatever I remember of my baseline. I was dragging this morning but definitely feel better now. This is the one time I'm not having a Ralph visit, so I won't know for sure if my Reds are low, but I'm wondering if I have been anemic, and now I'm coming around. I actually wonder if everything was suppressed, because I caught a very slight cold, which now seems to be departing.

I'm hoping the snow doesn't interfere with my visit to the DIEP dude on Friday. Rescheduling is such a drag.

We took Bobcat for his check-up today. He weighs in at 22 lbs. and 9 ounces. On the postcard reminder for his visit was a reminder for Charlie to have a fecal float. Could they come up with a more disgusting term? I am relieved to know that this just refers to a stool sample, and not a soda shoppe delicacy for dogs.

My family is running to watch the finale of America's Next Top Model, so I better sign off in order to get my intellectual stimulation for the evening.

December 18, 2007
DIEP thoughts

I had my visit with the DIEP dude on Friday. I had to wait an hour and a quarter before he even returned to the office, which is not a good thing for me (or anyone; I've never heard anyone wish for an hour wait for any kind of appointment). I was giving him another 10 minutes before leaving. This was the day after the Thursday snow storm, the storm of long rides home. I had driven an hour and a half to get a mile from my office when I called a friend who lived nearby (in Andover) and pleaded for shelter in her home. She and her husband graciously took me in, gave me tea by the fire, dinner, delightful company, and even assistance checking the roads before I headed for home at 9 p.m. I did not relish the possibility of being stuck in rush hour traffic on Friday.

So when he did come in, (DIEP DUDE) with the medical assistant and the fellow studying to do the DIEP, I was not my most outgoing self. I probably should have said something about the wait, as he did not, but at that point I just wanted to get on with it. I understand why people can be reluctant to complain to medical personnel that are responsible for their care. I am not usually hesitant to give feedback, either annoyed or pleased; but again, I didn't want to take the time.

We talked for a few minutes, and then he asked me to leave my robe on the chair and stand in front of the blue wall for photographs. I stood up and moved in front of the wall.

"You can leave your robe on the chair," he repeated.

Oh yeah.

In his world, it was commonplace to meet someone for three minutes, and then photograph her bare chest. In my world, not so much. I took a breath and draped the robe over the chair. He took mug shots; front view, each side, plus 45-degree angles. It was all very respectful and clinical, just not something I'm accustomed to doing.

When he returned (minus the medical assistant, who is female), he took his time explaining each of the reconstruction options, not just the DEIP. It was kind of like an historical tour through reconstruction options, starting with tissue expander/implant, moving to the tram and lat flaps, onto the DIEP, and then the glut flap.

The DIEP is unique in that it involves tissue from the abdominal area and blood vessels, but not the muscle. It is a long, delicate operation, because it takes time to separate out the tiny blood vessels from the abdominal muscles, lift them to the chest area, and connect them again. There is close monitoring the first 24 hours (at least hourly, if not more often), then the next four or five days in the hospital are the next critical level, and if you make it two weeks without complication, then you're probably good to go. It's another several weeks of recovery after that.

The tissue expander/implant route is less complicated up front. It's more straightforward without so many complicated issues surrounding blood vessels, etc. However, there is a greater chance of complications due to contracture, in which scar tissue forms around the tissue expander or implant, becoming tight and painful, and in some cases needing to be taken out altogether. With radiation, this can be up to 40 percent likely, which is quite a sizable chance.

I need to talk to my surgeon about this, because it seems that there is no way to hedge against these odds; the body either accepts the foreign object or it doesn't, in which case it starts to encapsulate and isolate the invading substance. I will need to have a serious chat with my bod in order to convince it that this is a welcome foreign object as opposed to the last foreign matter, which we excised as soon as we could. We've become used to dropping chemical bombs on everything in an effort to escort potential threats away efficiently and remind them that they are not welcome.

I'm still digesting this whole thing, as the DIEP is a much larger investment up front but involves less maintenance afterward. Because it is a person's own tissue, it expands or contracts along with any other tissue with weight gain or loss. The implant remains the same, while the rest of the body changes, which means that it may need to be swapped out or adjusted in 10 years or so. Or if we're going for matchsies, the other breast may need some adjustment. Actually, if I were to go the DIEP route, he told me he could create a new breast, but I would have to go down a cup size. This is not tragic, but it means an upfront adjustment on the other side. And this whole surgery should happen six months after my radiation if we want to play it safe (this offers the option to replace burned skin, if necessary).

When I can stop shivering and get out of my queasy feeling about the whole thing, I can consider my options. I'm still leaning toward the simpler upfront surgery. I have my last chemo treatment tomorrow and then no treatment until surgery, but appointments with each of my surgeons and with Hugs, pre-op work-up, MRI, mammogram, dentist. This was an intensely busy weekend, with Duke's work party 'til midnight, then up at six for Kate's gym meet (yes, in the snow), and Mom's amazing 80th birthday party later in the day. I haven't had the time to do a lot of reflecting, except when shoveling like mad.

So, DIEP dude did a great job of laying out the options, but apart from saying that he felt I'm a candidate, he couldn't say what my best option would be, because it is such a personal decision. Age, health, support system, age of kids, and lifestyle all factor in, and he can't possibly know which are my priorities. Only I can know that.

So off I go for my final glimpse of YEW. Whew! More from the other side.

December 21, 2007
Question of the Day (especially for New Yorkers)

In what way has chemo made me like a bus terminal? Think think think....

I have become a Port Authority! No groaning! More on my last Taxol later. Must Mall.

December 21, 2007
The Last of Yew

Wednesday was indeed the last round of Taxol. It has been so busy that I haven't really had time to digest this fact. I started to fill up, thinking about it, but was interrupted somehow in my reflection and haven't returned there. Which is fine. I will. Just one more piece of surreality in an otherwise surreal time.

I've got the acrid taste going, which means that I love that first cup of coffee and then can't stand the thought of it. Can't look at chocolate at the moment, either, which is a mixed blessing if ever there was one. Our house is abounding with the stuff, as the girls are bringing home delicacies of every description, and so am I. The Jolly Ranchers are appealing at the moment, or other strong flavors. So odd.

I have had fleeting numbness in two toes (probably hailing back to the sloth days) and occasionally my left cheek as well—the one on my face, thank you. We'll see if my head gets touchy.

I didn't seem to be as knocked out by the Benadryl this time. Maybe 'cause I had a stiffer cup of coffee, who knows. I was up at four yesterday, but slept in 'til five today, and I'm hoping the hour of shoveling today will help me to sleep in tomorrow.

I felt like Alice in Wonderland as I discovered a full pot of Duke's coffee in the bathroom this morning and decided to try it. Turns out it was 75 percent caf, stronger than my usual fare. So good all around that I got out there to shovel. And there was plenty. Eight to ten inches of snow, topped by an inch of ice, followed by another eight to ten inches of snow; a snow layer cake, with icing in between.

Off to the Cape on Sunday. We still don't have a tree up yet ourselves, which is a new record except for the year we moved here on Dec. 20, five years ago. Looks like tomorrow is the day....

I'm scheduled to the hilt with appointments in January, but am looking forward to some time with the fam, both on the Cape and in NYC this vacation. I'm sure I'll be writing again soon; looks like surgery will be on January 25, and as of now I'm staying with my original decision to do the tissue expander thing. We'll see if any of the number of conversations that I will have next month changes that.

May you all have peaceful, relaxing holidays, as much as possible. Again, I so appreciate your thoughts, ideas, love, and support. It is everything.

December 28, 2007

There is nothing quite so lovely as awakening to the mellifluous tones of your cat doing her level best to get the hairball from her stomach out onto your carpet. Right next to your bed. At 5 a.m. Daphne achieved this feat, and I was going to pull the "It's your turn" card, but realized that Duke was already downstairs. As I trudged down to find some paper towels, the kitchen light flipped on, and Duke and Bobcat both turned toward me with the same surprised expression on their faces. I had interrupted their snack ritual, and they were not expecting company. Even as annoyed as I was about my untimely cleaning chore, this sight totally tickled me. I found the towels, grabbed some kind of cleaner, and made my way back upstairs with a smile. I even managed to fall back asleep for a little while.

I'm hoping I'm beyond most of the weird side effects, like the taste thing and the tingly/numb thing (if I get it in my head, am I a numb-skull?). My taste buds have definitely returned to normal. Kate warned me that all the chocolate that had held no interest would now be tempting me. Oh my god! We have dark chocolate, milk chocolate, white chocolate with peppermint, truffles, assorted chocolates, chips, even a tiny chocolate mouse from Burdick's! Where before I had been completely oblivious to them, now I see them peering down at me, declaring the holiday bounty. Scary.

Most of the tingly is gone, but there's still some occasionally in my toes and face. I am glad that I don't have any more chemo treatments, and that I don't have to prepare myself for the odd physical events that follow them.

More than one person has suggested some sort of send-off for Dolly. While I appreciate and totally believe in the power of ritual, this feels like too much focus for me right now. I am needing to look beyond and remind myself that this is just a stop along the way, with much more to look forward to, in the most positive sense of the word. If I hover too much around the loss it makes me anxious, and that is not a useful stopping point. Maybe I will feel differently in the weeks to come, but at least for now I prefer not to set that up. We'll see. In the highly individual aspect of this thing, there is room for each person to choose what feels best, what makes one feel whole.

We spent a few days on the Cape around Christmas. Just before we left, I went to retrieve the Sunday paper so there would be room for

Monday's mail. The paper was in the snow, and in the mailbox was a card from Sheila with an angel ornament engraved with the words, "I said a prayer for you today."

I was touched and taken off guard. There are points where it's possible to anticipate an emotional reaction and times when this is not predictable. This was one of those. I came inside, hung the ornament on the tree, and felt that it would be a positive reminder of this Christmastime. Then I became teary, because I do not want people to have to worry about me. I don't want to worry about myself, or need special care or consideration. But this is where things are right now, and I am fortunate to have such a caring circle. Even when I am not aware of it, and perhaps especially when I am not aware of it, the circle moves around, sending its messages in ways large and small so that I know I am anything but alone.

I am humbled once again and misty when I bring our bags out to the truck. Duke has been feeling pressed to get going but stops to pause and catch a few tears that have been released by this kindness.

The Cape brings its own mixture of fun and struggle, but we gather and eat, and the cousins bake chocolate chip cookies. Val, my mother-in-law, was in pain as she struggled with the last stages of multiple myeloma, and we all realized that this would be our last Christmas together. Mark flew in from his scheduled time in Vancouver to be present for Val's favorite holiday. Charlie (Mr. Dog) always insists on a walk at some ungodly hour when we're there, and I volunteer the first morning. I love walking there, so near the ocean, even if it's a tad chilly at 6 a.m. When we return, I doze and dream that I am being driven off road in some kind of jeep. Part of this may come from the book I had been reading, which was taking place in part in the African bush. Or maybe I feel like I have been far off the beaten path.

At some point I realize we need to get back to the road, but the brush is too dense, and I don't know how we're going to get there. I don't know who the driver is, but we are suddenly airborne, rising over the vegetation. I am exhilarated; I love being in the air. I can see all around. I was woken at this point, but I am still thrilled to have spent some time lifted off the ground. I'm not sure what it all means, but it has been a long time since I have had a flying dream, and it always feels freeing. Maybe I will try to get back there to finish the dream.

Gale and Duke both encouraged me to consider the DIEP, to think about the long term and not be as concerned with the upfront investment if it will be better in the long run. I will think about it some more after this weekend in NYC. There have been too many areas of my life crowding for attention, but once the holidays are past, more space will open up.

For now, I'm looking forward to RENT, visiting, and being in a New York state of mind. Happy New Year!!!!

December 31, 2007

Hoppy Newt Year!

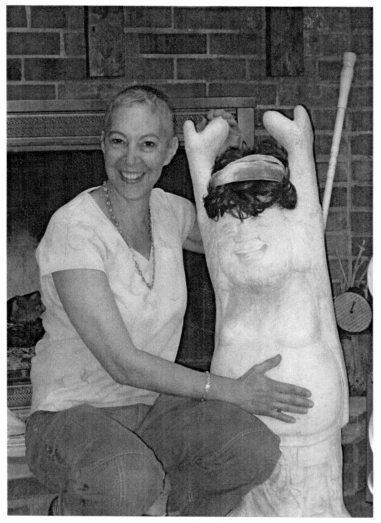

Christmas Day 2007

Chapter 3

Moving Mountains

January 8, 2008
On to the Next....

We're into the second week in January, and my surgery is now a little more than two weeks off. My pre-op tests—EKG, blood work, mammogram, and MRI—were all fine. The phlebotomist (phlebotomy recapitulates phylogeny, or some such scientific bastardization...) was amazing; I barely even felt the needle. The person at the MRI, on the other hand, had the disadvantage of using a larger needle, because it needed to deliver some dye at the end of the test. This required a couple of pokes, and some digging around to land an accepting vein. And I had become so cavalier about these things.

Although I'm pleased the results of all these tests were fine, it is not terribly consoling, as they were also fine before my lumpectomy in July. Certainly, it is a good thing for there not to be something concerning that showed up, but I was definitely not expecting that there would be.

Anyway, we'll see what Hugs has to say tomorrow. I'm squeezing him in between a walk (hopefully) and a massage. And I'm finally going to use that gift certificate from Duke on Valentine's Day last year.

I'm starting to consider the surgery and prepare for it in my way.

A client asked if I was nervous. I said yes, and she followed up with, "Is it the surgery that you're worried about? Have you ever had surgery?"

I realized that I'm not too worried about the surgery. I know now that I react fine to the anesthesia (except that I am incurably chatty once I surface, and will pay a visit to Loopyville's roller coaster the next day, most likely.) The pain is definitely manageable, and in the long run, my life is going to remain mostly the same. I will be walking around as soon as I can after surgery, building up to my 3-mile loop. I'll start biking in the spring and swimming in the summer. I will still be able to enjoy the myriad things I find fun.

Yes, absolutely there will be some tender moments with my Breasty Business, and the bandages, and the drain game, but at least I'm familiar with the thing. I have visits to look forward to (with people other than my medical team!), and some time off from work. I'll be able to read some more of the books that I have been given, both for the holidays, and through your kindness. And I will be one step closer to finished with my triathlon.

My plan is to take two weeks off from work. I think this is realistic; I have appointments with my surgeons this week and next, and can ask some more questions so that I can anticipate as best as I can what to expect. There can be no total preparation for the loss, and the change in appearance. I can only do what I can do in this regard. Verdad?

I put my wig on backward a few weeks ago. I can now say that I know what I would look like with eyes in the back of my head. I had not intended to do it, but I just grabbed the critter off its stand and popped it on. Not so very different, really. I wonder if I could fool the kids into thinking I was looking the other way.

New Year's was relaxing. Duke was in Falmouth, Gale was at Anne's, and Kate had a couple of friends over. We played games, they watched a movie, we rang in the New Year with Dick Clark, and had sparkling cider in champagne glasses. The next day was more games, fun in the snow, and finishing my book. Our time in NYC was lovely as well;

fulfilled Gale's promise to Kate to see Rent for her 13th birthday.

More once I'm on the other side of my next round of visits. As usual, I didn't realize how much was ready to pop out until I sat down to dash off a note (it's kind of like going to the supermarket for one thing and coming back $100 later).

January 9, 2008
Emerson

I don't know what they were selling at Emerson Hospital today, but I had to leave the parking lot, then re-enter and stalk a little boy and his dad in order to get a parking spot (they were unaware, don't worry). I was entertained by the fact that there was a bowl of Hershey's kisses at the check-in for my appointment with Hugs. Very appropriate.

Nothing new to report from him, except that he thought it was six to eight weeks post-op that I start radiation; I thought three, and I'm glad that I had the beat on this one. I wouldn't want to wait around that long. He was encouraging about my surgery, saying that sometimes it needs to be delayed because someone is so depleted from chemo. He feels that I'm going into it strong, and that I should not take this for granted. He's right, and I am appreciative of how well I feel.

Went from there to my massage, which was great, of course. I need to have a masseuse on staff, clearly. And I'm willing to share. The table was heated. Just what someone with breakthrough heat needs.

Plastic man on Friday. Do you think plastic man has a rubber duck?

January 11, 2008
Plastics!!

Plastic Doc helped clarify a few issues, and agreed with me that I can always do the DIEP later on, but if I don't do the tissue expander now, it is most likely not a possibility. It will be partially expanded at the time of the surgery next week, and he will continue to expand it over the next several weeks, up until and possibly overlapping with the beginning of radiation. He can't put an implant in right away because I'll need the firmer tissue expander to resist the tightening effects of the radiation, and because it is not clear yet how much of the skin will be saved from the surgery. I'm hoping to stay the same size, but we'll see how it goes.

I expressed my concerns about the complication rate, and he agreed that it is higher with the radiation, but that these complications may include small changes that need to be made, or small infections, and that he has only had to actually take the expander out because of contracture for one person.

I kept asking if there was something that I could do to be helpful in this process. For people like me, who are do-ers, it is helpful to feel like there is some contribution to make, to be more than just a recipient of care.

He said that I'm already a non-smoker, then thought a little more and said, "You can be patient. It will take several months for this whole process, and at least six months before we can put in the implant, so remember that the way it is after surgery is not how it will be in the end. We can create a better reconstruction with a few smaller surgeries than we can with one big one."

This is key for me to remember in terms of my expectations. I need to not get stuck in the now. This is a more fluid process than I had originally conceived. As much as I want it to be over, I cannot shortcut the steps.

That's why it is so good for me to have lots of fun distractions, be they work, play, visits, whatever. I need to continue living my life, and I need to make sure there is enough room to accommodate time for my Breasty Business. It's just that sometimes, like now, it takes up a little more space than I'd like.

Plastic Doc also said that I will probably be in the hospital a day or two, and that the Visiting Nurse Assistant will visit. I'll go home with a local anesthetic pump thingy that they can take out after a few days.

I think that's about it. Some more info after Tuesday's visit with Cat Woman (my *general* surgeon who will deliver *colonels* of info about my not-so-*major* surgery). Cat woman because she has a number of them besides the one who visits in the office.

January 18, 2008
On Deck....

I sat in the waiting room for my surgeon, looking through the stack of photo albums of the gingerbread mansions she produces each year. I had read about them in our paper, but never actually seen them. Each little album shows the stages of production of these wildly colorful creations, crafted as carefully and intricately as...a surgeon might. On the walls are animals she's photographed on safari. When I am shown into her office, sure enough, there is a photo on the corner of her desk of a tiny cat curled up in her bed.

We discuss the surgery. She asks questions about my visit with the Plastic Guy, and it is clear that the two of them need to have another conversation, and also that she will follow through with this quickly. She confirmed that I will likely be in the hospital one night. She doesn't want me hanging around there if I don't need to. I will probably have a pair of drains that will stay in about a week. Last time it went longer, but that is not necessarily predictive. I keep trying to rely on history to provide information, but this proves to be an inaccurate measure of what to expect. But we're talking a matter of a few days difference. She is pleased with the MRI and mammo results.

So: I am all cleared and ready to go for next Friday.

On Wednesday, I hit the slopes with Susan at Wachusett. What a treat! I was actually surprised there wasn't more snow, but they must have had some freezing rain when we got our 14 inches on Monday. I love it there; being outside, the exercise, the company, and skiing itself. Someday I will go several days in a row and really improve. In the meantime, it is still fab.

For the second time this week, Kate encouraged me to take a bath rather than a shower. I'm trying out some of the bath fizzes we have collected. Is this bathological? Whatever, it's a fun part of my relaxation regimen. It's all contributing to my going into Friday as peaceful and even as I can. And then I get two whole weeks off from work!

I told my surgeon that I had promised my family I wouldn't shovel for a month, and she looked horrified and said immediately, "Oh, no, you can't shovel!"

She was clearly not appreciating that I was joking. Of course I'm not going to shovel. What, hasn't she been following my e-mails? I will have to pin down one of the surgeons about activity level. Each deferred to the other about this. Polite, but not effective.

Duke will go to the Cape today, and I'm hoping to go early tomorrow. Our hearts continue to be with his dad and stepmom through these difficult stages.

January 21, 2008
Wicked shirt

In my enthusiasm for the song *Defying Gravity* when we saw *Wicked* a few years ago, I bought tee shirts for the girls and myself. The first time I pulled mine out and saw the song title across my chest I giggled and wondered whether that little joke was intentional. It had been in my dresser for awhile, and I just came across it the other day. Well, I am about to create more reason to defy gravity. It's so odd what occurs to me—maybe they should hand out Defy Gravity shirts to everyone going in for reconstruction.

I continue to feel well. My own deal is minuscule compared to my mother-in-law's transition…she is showing amazing grace and clarity, and I see the circle of love and support around her.

I remain humbled by my own incredible circle, and feel completely surrounded and held. It helps me feel calm and ready. I want music in my room at Emerson. I want them to ask who is singing in there. I was singing to the Bangles on the ski slope. I was singing Joan Armatrading's *Show Some Emotion.* You should feel free to sing, too.

January 22, 2008

———————— *Forwarded message* —————-

*From: **Ana Martinez***
Date: Jan 21, 2008 2:28 PM
Subject: Meg's Pre-and-post Surgery
Hello All.

Duke and I have chatted about what we believe our most favorite snow-shoveling Punster Queen will need during her pre-and post-surgery time. Instinctively, we each know that the real response to "What does Meg need during this time?" is simply, "to get out of her way." But how much fun would that be, really?

Instead, we ask that you email Meg Ellen Sperber Stafford your best puns, reports of the absurd, good YouTube links, or—if you're really mature—well wishes and loving support. She has so enjoyed her emails to you, updating you on her process and progress, but she does crave a little "pre-and post-" text from us.
Best,
Ana

January 22, 2008

From: Joni Coleman Magurn
Date: 2008/01/22 Tue PM 01:11:25 CST
Subject: Helping Meg

Dear Friends of Meg,

Jill Chick and I (also Buddies of Meg [BOMs] :) would like to enlist your help in making Meg's road to recovery following her surgery a bit less rocky. We are asking for volunteers to provide dinner for the Stafford family each night beginning on Saturday the 26th. Jill and I will create a calendar and act as contact points to coordinate the meals. We are hoping that eliminating the work involved in providing dinner each night gives a little relief to an already overburdened family.

If you would like to help, please email me and let me know which night works best for you. At that time, I will let you know the particulars (dietary guidelines, drop off info, etc.). Thank you in advance for your generosity in making life a bit easier for our friend.

Joni Coleman Magurn

January 24, 2008
Launching Pad

I had a massage yesterday, which was divine. This one was even better than the last; somehow I was able to relax more deeply, and the masseuse seemed more tuned in. When I went to pull out my gift card, I could not find it. Yes, Missy Organized somehow misplaced the card she had pulled out the day before. Anyway, I paid with my credit card, and they will resurrect the gift card, and I can use it at another time. Isn't that handy? I'll have to go another time. Dang.

The situation with my mother-in-law is amazingly still unfolding. I spent last Saturday in Falmouth; Duke was there the whole weekend. The girls and I drove down on Tuesday to say goodbye, essentially. Mark, our dear friend, and Duke's stepbrother, asked if I was feeling upstaged.

Well, yes, actually, yes I am, I replied. As it should be.

Death trumps any other issue, and this is her time. She is a model as she moves into her transition. In my selfishness I had been anxious, worried that I would not be able to attend the service, but this will not be the case. As I wrote my last e-mail, talking about singing in my hospital room, I learned that Val had requested that the girls and I sing at her service. We are honored by her request and have found a song that fits. We are sad that we cannot be in Falmouth now, but relieved to know that there are others there to be with Val, and with Doug. We will be there as soon as we can.

Right now, we need to focus on being here and getting to tomorrow afternoon. My plan is to be up in my room. It's not a complicated plan, but it's helpful to be looking through to the other side.

Okay, deep breath.

I feel all the good stuff coming my way, and it will carry me through. I know it. Time to change out of my work clothes and get ready for bed. I have a great silly book—one of Louise Rennison's books about Georgia Nicholson. My favorite title of hers was *Away Laughing on a Fast Camel*.

From Betsy:

Hi, Meg—if the cosmos are cooperating, you should be feeling a wave of somethin' from the south (support? smothering affection?). You are uppermost in our minds and hearts day and night!!

We continue to be awed by and grateful for the opportunity to be a tiny part of your journey. While this is certainly secondary to all else, I thought it was worthy of mention (as maybe you haven't yet realized it): your sharing all of this has already changed each of us on the receiving end in ways that will only be fully realized over time: as we live our lives and face our own personal challenges as well as how we're able to help— in both small and large ways—those we love face challenges.

I don't know if you've ever seen this essay by Ralph Waldo Emerson. A dear friend gave it to me years ago when I was going through a difficult time. I just came across it again—you are the banyan of the forest.

COMPENSATION

The compensations of calamity are made apparent to the understanding
also, after long intervals of time. A fever, a mutilation, a cruel disappointment,
a loss of wealth, a loss of friends, seems at the moment unpaid loss, and
unpayable. But the sure years reveal the deep remedial force that underlies
all facts. The death of a dear friend, wife, brother, lover, which seemed nothing
but privation, somewhat later assumes the aspect of a guide of genius; for it
commonly operates revolutions in our way of life, terminates an epoch of
infancy or of youth which was waiting to be closed, breaks up a wonted occu-
pation, or a household, or style of living, and allows the formation of new ones
more friendly to the growth of character.

It permits or constrains the formation of new acquaintances and the
reception of new influences that prove of the first importance to the next years;
and the man or woman who would have remained a sunny garden-flower,
with no room for its roots and too much sunshine for its head, by the falling of
the walls and the neglect of the gardener it is made the Banyan of the forest,
yielding shade and fruit to wide neighborhoods of men.

— Ralph Waldo Emerson, Poems of Ralph Waldo Emerson, T. Y.
    Crowell (NY), 1965

Xoxoxo,

Betsy

PS: Now, to be true to my stupid side (and I'm putting myself out there revealing this!), if you're looking for a chuckle, go to YouTube and search for "Flight of the Conchords, Business Time." I have to admit, embarrassingly enough, that I fell out of my chair.

From Duke: Meg's Doing Very Nicely, Thanks

Hi, All,

Just a quick note then I'm off to visit with herself. According to the "Plastic Guy," the operation went very well with no complications. She was literally doing laps around the sixth floor by 5 p.m. Not quite at her sub-jog pace, but not far off. I think perhaps the anesthesia was still providing some comfort. I just spoke to her, she is more sore today.

I want to thank you all, from my heart, for your well wishes, positive energy, and your loving kindnesses. Meg and I feel swaddled in loving support as we make our way on this challenging journey. It is the brilliant light on this unexpected path.

I'm sure you will hear from her directly later today or tomorrow. We expect to bring her home this afternoon.

Love to All,
Duke

On a sad note, my stepmother passed away last night after a long battle with cancer. Yesterday afternoon, Meg asked that Val be given the message that the operation had gone well, and she was fine. Though she was not conscious, I know the message got through. It seemed over the last week or so she was holding on to life, not wanting to let go. She passed away quietly several hours after my brother Mark gave her the message. When I shared this with my brother Bob last night, he said she was waiting to take all the cancer with her. Val was a loving friend, companion, and challenging intellect to my mother and father. They all met in college. Sometime after my mother passed away in 1988, Val and Dad were married. He was twice blessed to share his life, 50+ years, with two remarkable women.

January 26, 2008
I'm Baaaaa aaaaack!!

Arrived home around one today. Plastic Doc was in charge, and as soon as he saw me sitting in the chair, he announced that I'm obviously doing well and ready to go. Within the hour, I was on the road with Duke and Kate.

He gave me a passel of prescriptions...three different pain meds to try. My first nurse in the hospital was very hesitant to give me any pain medication because I have this pump attached for the first three to four days. She said that what I was experiencing was probably muscle soreness.

SO?!

I just had surgery involving the removal of a lot of tissue, moving of muscle, and the placement of a foreign object in my body. OF COURSE I WOULD BE SORE!! That's what the pain medication is for, for Christ's sake!

I finally convinced her to give me some last night and slept soundly from midnight to four, then dozed for a few hours before turning on my light and reading. The morning nurse was not so hesitant, and the Doc said that I should definitely be on oral pain meds every three to four hours. The local anesthetic pump is an aid, not the whole deal. When I take it, I can walk around doing everything that doesn't involve lifting heavy things. I feel pretty good.

I'm trying out Percocet now, and I have to say, it does not seem to make me quite so loopy. Same with the Dilaudid. Can't do this quite like a wine tasting (I guess it's supposed to eliminate whine testing...), but I'll definitely give them all a try.

The pump will be finished on Monday, and hopefully Duke is up to pulling it out (once I am loaded up on one of my pain variety meds). The drain will be removed by the doc on Friday, and then I'll see Resciniti (the General) the following week. They were both very complimentary of the other (the docs, that is) which is cute. So nice they get to chat during the surgery.

I'm relieved to be home and have this stage of the triathlon behind me. I know there is more to come; I haven't yet taken a look under the bandages; that can wait a few days. But I am glad to have emerged feeling as well as I do. I'm not quite ready for my 3-mile loop, but it does feel good to be able to be vertical and have something more interesting than the hospital North 6 to look at.

I felt you with me. Last night before I went to sleep, I lay there just thinking about everyone.

Duke's brother Bob came to visit Duke during my surgery. I had asked Bob to contact Mark so he could let Val, my mother-in-law, know that my surgery went well. When I learned today that she died a few hours after that I felt a mix of emotions. Susan had suggested that perhaps she was waiting to know that everything had gone well with me. I do believe that people wait for particular events, but it had not occurred to me that it could have to do with me. Who knows whether it did or not. Even the possibility blows me away.

More soon, but two silly things. One really bad hospital term: the urine and stool hat. It is a plastic inverted hat shaped device which fits in the toilet so that it can intercept the bodily fluids before hitting the porcelain. It's used to measure "output" so that they know a person's plumbing is in order, but what an image.

Also, I noticed the other day that I had the tiniest, teeniest little bit of bed head! Yes, the peach fuzz is on the move. At the rate of a quarter of an inch a month, it could be awhile before I can create the Annie Lennox look, but I'm looking forward to the return of the hair. And I'm relieved about the end of the port, which was removed during the same surgery in which Dolly exited. The incision hurts right now, but that should be much better in a couple of days, and I no longer have that big vein look on the right side of my neck. (Okay, that was a third thing.)

Signing off for now, ready to watch the first of many movies in these next couple of weeks. Let's hope I'm awake longer than the opening scene...any recommendations for others?

January 28, 2008
Day 4 Lore

Well, here we are, visiting Day 4. I have been warned that healing is not linear, and that I should expect that days three and four may bring more reactions to the anesthesia, pain, etc. If it's one thing I should have learned by now, it is that history is not always a predictor for how things go, and that as above, healing does not happen in a straight, predictable line.

Anyway, I am very mobile, and am testing out my three pain meds, trying to figure out which one is best. So far, I have been alternating them in no particular order, and my only observations are that Vicodin seems the strongest, and also makes me the most loopy or light headed. Dilaudid seems the gentlest, and leaves me with a relatively recognizable brain. I guess that leaves Percocet somewhere in-between. They all dry me up like a desert plant, so I need copious amounts of fluid and fruit to keep up. I seem to get a little shivery when the pain meds run out, or as I'm realizing right now, it may also be coinciding with running low on fuel. I've been trying not to overeat, so it may be that I need little bits more frequently.

As promised, I have not lifted a shovel or a laundry basket. I shocked my family by sitting for two, yes two movies yesterday, plus two episodes of *Project Runway*. I did catch a little snooze during *Spiderman 3* (which is fine, it's not a great film), but I was capable of all that viewing without having to bike-ride first.

People have encouraged me to milk it and take advantage of having the fam do things. Partly this is good, but I like being able to do things, and it makes me feel more normal to unload the dishwasher or fold some laundry. I can't drive, and we are sooooo grateful for the meals on wheels that are providing not only dinner but spillover into the next day's lunches. The silly little house chores that I *can* do help me feel like I'm contributing. Call me kooky, but that's what works for me.

"Duke Couture" has returned, this time with the corduroy and flannel collection. They're perfect—soft, button down, and big enough to get around the pump and drain. We'll go down to the Cape for the services for Val this weekend. I think there will be a lot of people there from various times in Doug's and Val's lives, and it will be a lot to take in.

Bob has suggested that I wear a sling so that people know not to hug me. It is very frustrating not to hug people, because this is exactly what I want to do, but can't. The sling idea may be a good one, or I'll have to think of some alternative. Being there will make her death real, which at this point is slightly abstract, given the distance. We've been kind of distracted, and I'm sure the real part of missing her will be magnified once we're there.

There is a lot of emotion flying around right now, and I'm betting that we are not aware of the toll. It is completely tempered by the support in every way from all of you. Hey, if I can blame my activity level on you, maybe my family won't complain when I'm up bopping around.

I've decided to keep cards and things in my Rocket Dog box. I love saying it out loud. Try it once with emphasis and feeling:

Rocket Dog.

It's cool, huh? Makes you feel good.

I'm taking each thing as it comes, and am concentrating on the healing, keeping my body relaxed so that my muscles don't tense up and hurt. I'm worried about the next phase, which will involve a peek at Driscoll's and Resciniti's handiwork, because as much as I have a high pain tolerance, I have a very low squeam tolerance, and it doesn't take much to make me feel faint. That will be a whole other wave of emotion. For now, bring on the movies.

January 29, 2008
Roller Coaster

I thought I had it outwitted. Closing in on the end of Day 4, pirouetting my way through the day, I had become a little bit smug. By keeping on moving, I was sure that I had escaped whatever could be dished out. How wrong I was.

There waiting for me at 9 p.m., when I was really tired, whipping out from behind the den couch with a flourish, was the Anesthesia Rollercoaster. Some of you will remember this phenomenon from the summer, when I experienced the next day departure of anesthesia in an irrational flood of tears and laughter rolled into one bizarre hour. I think it waited longer this time because it was a longer surgery, requiring more anesthesia, and also because it was aiming for the element of surprise as it lurked around the edges of the computer or in back of the fridge.

I sat down on the couch in the den to join Duke in a little relaxation and TV viewing. Gale was off at a friend's and Kate had gone up for a post-gymnastics shower. It started with the tears. I was itching from where the pump attaches and where the drain is stitched in, and wanted to be cleaned up where the blood seeped through along the lines for the pump. Driscoll had seen these and was unconcerned, but it couldn't be thoroughly cleaned because some of it was under the tape holding the apparatus in place.

I didn't want to burden Duke with this. He has been through enough, and I didn't want to make one more demand. Hence the tears. He sat in front of me and asked what was wrong. I started to explain through my blubbering, and then we heard a whistling sound. Looking around, we realized that it was emanating from Bobcat's nose, as he dozed. We both burst out laughing.

And then I was crying again, because I still hadn't resolved the cleaning up issue, and I was tired of it. And then Bobcat whistled, and we were laughing again. Back and forth.

Duke handed me some tissues and held the little wastebasket out so I could take aim for it (scoring twice in a row, I might add). Bob shifted positions so that his head was on my leg and he was on his back with his four paws all draped together. He looked ridiculous, producing more laughter. Even though we both knew what was happening, I was utterly helpless to control it. I wanted to just cry it all out so that I could relax, but I couldn't because something would strike me as funny.

Blessedly, as in the past, the whole ordeal lasted less than an hour. I was ready to finally get up, but then I didn't want to because Bobcat had shifted again and looked so completely comfortable I didn't want to leave him. Part of it was the sucker part of me, but the other part wanted to absorb his utter relaxation and ability to melt into my leg, the couch, whatever was near him. I know I've talked about this before, but his superior relaxation skills continue to astound me. His unquestionable knowledge that everything is as it should be, his continual living in what Duke calls the Comfort Zone is very appealing right now. I did get up, and the rest of his body just poured into the blanket on the couch, so clearly I didn't need to worry about him. It was the comfort he was providing me that I was holding on to.

I thought about removing the pump myself today, but both Duke and Kate asked me not to, and I know they're right. That's an adventure for later, when people are home. We visit Driscoll at the crack of rush-hour on Thursday and Resciniti next week. I was hoping for drain removal this week, but we'll see. I would rather have it through the weekend if necessary than have another Dolly issue somewhere.

Today is my first day home without people here. I usually cherish time to myself, and know I will enjoy it, but I think that some company will also be a good thing. First, taxes. Everything in balance (not that that applies to taxes…).

January 29, 2008
Pumped!!

Not! Duke removed the tiny twin catheters without a hitch in about one minute flat. Now I need to recalibrate my pain meds. Let's hope the drain removal is both soon and as smooth. I think I am now feeling the insertion site.

January 30, 2008
Play Dates

Okay, so I'm counting on you guys to help me out with my avoidance around some of the work I've brought home. I'm finding that I have a fair amount of energy (there's a surprise), and that I'm really wanting to see people. One of the silver linings (or chartreuse and fuchsia) has to be that I get to see people who I don't normally get to see. So come out and play!! I know, I'm supposed to be resting and all that, and visiting IS resting. Otherwise, I'm figuring out how to bring down a load of laundry without picking up the whole basket and stuff like that. I was good at movies while the girls were still home…maybe I just need some new ones here in the house.

I'm not cooking too much, although I'm a wizard in the reheating department, and I know how to pull out those pots and pans without even breaking anything (of myself or other dishes…).

I have started saving Vicodin for the night, because it knocks me on my butt and bed is a good place to be when this happens. Am I repeating myself repeating myself? Now I just alternate between the other two during the day. I still need the same amount, because with the pump no longer helping locally (as opposed to in California), I need to keep up with the new sensations that are coming through. I might even need a tad more at first. I have to talk myself into it because I really don't want to increase anything. I have been told that I do talk to myself already. (Thank you, Gale. I guess I respond aloud to e-mail some-times…so I am not actually talking to myself, but to you, or to junk mail.) Anyway, I digress. I'm working out the pain thing, and I'm really pretty comfortable for the most part. And I've asked for assistance in changing the beds. How's that for progress?

I feel better now that I've got that out. After all, how can I expect you to distract me, and stop me from charging ahead with my work homework if you didn't know it was there to be avoided? Now that you know, you should feel free to come in and rip it to shreds, or anything else that might accidentally happen if I leave it in the middle of the driveway, or on top of the doormat. Thanks so much.

February 1, 2008
Tough Day

This is where this thing is really more for me than for you. Yesterday was complicated, and I need to sort it out, because I need to be ready for the next wave.

Duke took me to Driscoll's, where we arrived at 7 a.m. for our 7:30 appointment, because we happened to hit a day on Route 128 where there was relatively little traffic. This allowed me to drape myself over Duke for awhile because taking the Vicodin at midnight means that I am beyond loopy into zomboidland if I'm waking up at 5:30 a.m. Driscoll was very kind and gentle when removing the bandages, and pleased with how things are progressing, although he said it was too early to remove the drain, and this will happen at my return trip on Monday. With my lymph nodes gone, I have a compromised drainage system, kind of like Route 16 as opposed to Route 495 (and I have often studied the drainage systems on these roads…).

I made a point of looking away, because I figure the more time I give the surgery to look less bruised and swollen, the easier it will be to bear when I do peek. Except that I caught a little glimpse out the corner of my eye. It looked like the pictures he had shown me. And it's not me. Except that it is.

I'm digesting this and gradually getting used to it. It didn't fully hit until I was telling Susan on the phone. Duke overheard my teary voice as he was getting ready to head out to a walk-through for work and decided to take the rest of the day off after that. He came home with movies. It took us the rest of the afternoon and evening to get through one of them because of various interruptions, both welcome and not (and I have to watch it again, because this is when I chose to nap…)!

Later in the afternoon, I got a call from Resciniti telling me that the pathology from the surgery showed that there was one more 5-mm spot that was found deeper in the breast tissue, closer but not touching the chest wall, and that it was a good choice to both have the surgery, and to have radiation that is soon to be scheduled.

I was literally being woken from sleep and so did not think to ask questions like "were the cells compromised or not" or "what are the implications for the other breast" etc., which I will address with her next week, and with Hugs. Although it freaked us out, George was not concerned by this news; he was more pleased that the margin was clear. In some ways it was not news. We had already known that there were other sites. But since the MRI was clean, this brought home the fact that it isn't a perfect test, which raises *more* questions.

There is nothing immediate to be done. I need to get through the weekend before addressing it more aggressively. And it is only I who can truly decide, once I have some more information, how important it is to consider a prophylactic mastectomy of Dolly's Pardner.

Whew! I had been working hard to get our tax stuff in order so that we can get the FAFSA done (Brown University's deadline is today), and heard from our accountant at 10 p.m. last night. We owe the feds $2100. Great. How the hell did this happen?! We're so careful. I'm glad it was last night and not today that this final piece of joy was delivered, because today is a new day, and I have more energy and a firmer conviction that we will deal with whatever comes, that we will work it out. If the challenges could please just space themselves out a little better, that would be very nice. We are going to need some major play time in between.

Okay, I think that's it for the moment. Driscoll suggested I get some good sports bras. I take this to mean that he's very optimistic about my getting back to my sports (or that this is how one becomes a good sport). Also, I just picked up an e-mail that the girls' school is going to close at noon. Is there that much weather about to happen?!!

February 4, 2008
Weekend

Val's service was intense, personal, and deeply satisfying. It was held in the Quaker Meeting House in Falmouth, a beautiful, simple, light-filled place with just enough room to hold the roughly 100 people who attended. Doug's sister Nancy started us off by explaining that anyone who wished to could speak, and that after a moment of silence, she would start.

Val was raised Catholic, but was not practicing, and although some family members had some doubts about having a service without a Mass, Doug was clear that this is what she wanted. Nancy read the poem that Val had read for Virginia, (Doug's first wife and Val's best friend) when she died, and truly for everything there is a season. Doug spoke next, and each of Val's three children, some of her grandchildren, and sons-/daughters-in-law, someone from her work life, and people from various other times and parts of her life.

The girls and I were joined by Mark's girlfriend, Laurie, when we sang *The Book I'm Not Reading* by Patti Larkin. Val was a voracious reader, and there was always another book to add to her shelf. It was the right blend of something that was about her, had an easy-going melody, and was easy to harmonize. After 10 minutes of practice, it was clear that Laurie was meant to make us a vocal quartet. It felt good to contribute to the service in this way. Together, we all painted a picture of who Val was, her importance to so many, and the varied contributions she made to people on numerous continents. I always learn about someone at a memorial service, and this was no exception.

The hug thing turned out to not be an issue. Most people who know me were careful. Those who didn't were not inclined to randomly give me a bear hug (shocking though that may be).

One person who was in an in-between category gave a nice hug, and I involuntarily blurted out "Easy!"

"Nice to see you, too," he replied. Interesting what you hear when there's a lot of ambient noise (and there's a little bit of a hearing problem, I found out later).

It is difficult to see so many people who are hurting, yet at the same time it is a comfort to be around people who cared about and knew Val across so many contexts. There is no substitute for the time it will take to heal.

Today (moving on to Monday) I paid another visit to Dr. Driscoll, and the nurse took out my drain. Yea!! I can see clearly now, the drain is gone. Don't ask me what vision has to do with the drain (or rain) being gone, but evidently it should now be improved. He's going away for two weeks, and wants everything sewn up (so to speak) before he goes away, so there's one small area that is a little slower in healing that he's tempted to incise and re-stitch just to make sure it's all set.

"No big deal," he said. Just a little half hour procedure right here in the office.

Part of this is also driven by what the radiation plans are, which are yet to be determined. Ah yes, just a little procedure. Well, I would prefer not to have it if I don't have to, thanks very much. No big deal, just a few stitches, but that means a few more days' discomfort, and healing, and no big deal if that's what's necessary, but please. So I will diligently put hydrogen peroxide on it in an effort to coax it into a higher healing gear. And I'll call my radiation gal.

The secretary scheduled my visit for 3:30 on Friday. What do they think? That I'm just hanging around going to appointments? Waiting for rush hour? Oh yeah. That is pretty much the deal these two weeks. That's why those movies are so key. I have a good stack now, and books I'm not reading.

Last week was an interesting mail convergence. Sympathy cards, get well cards, every one of them welcome. There was one flower delivery.

"These are for you," I announced to Duke. "From something or other Insulation."

He looked more closely. "Nope, they're for you," he countered. "From one of the contractors we do work with."

What a pathetic statement that we're having trouble sorting the mail because of all that's going on. It was at least an objective confirmation that if we're a little confused, we can blame something other than medication.

This is a big relief because I'm mostly down to Tylenol now. Except that I took a Percocet just to preempt any post-visit discomfort. Now I'm sleepy. I'm going to see what happens when I get horizontal. Many of you may have tried this experiment. It's something you're supposed to try at home. I'll let you know how it goezzzzzzzzz....

February 9, 2008
Too Much

I hardly know where to start. First off, let me say that my healing continues. After my Percocet fog on Monday, I have stayed away from prescribed sleepiness and have stuck with Tylenol when necessary. My energy level has increased daily, and I've been trying to rest when I need it. I did drive to the polls on Tuesday and to get my oil changed.

I saw my general surgeon (not the Surgeon General) on Thursday; she took one look and asked to see me in June after my next mammo. We had quite a long chat, especially for her. She said that lobular invasive cancer (including the most recent spot found in the pathology from surgery) does not put Parton at greater risk. It would be the presence of LCIS that would (this is a marker that I do not have). The risk is there because of Dolly's experience.

I still need to speak to Hugs to ask more about what the cells looked like that were found, etc., but at least so far, the pathology does not seem to hold new information in terms of what to do next, or any greater concern than was there before. I have some more thoughts on that, but have not fully digested them, and so cannot say anything comprehensible yet.

I saw Driscoll on Friday, and he did a little cleaning to the spot that he had some concerns about and handed me a couple of tiny bacitracin samples. He told me to keep cleaning it, but that he felt like it looked great and would be fine for radiation, which should begin in a couple of weeks. As he ripped open a packet of instruments, I asked him for a moment. He stopped, and I took a deep breath so that I could relax. Again, this was a little, 5-minute procedure for him and the nurse, but I am not accustomed to having someone poking around on my chest and feeling not so much pain as pressure. It takes me a minute to get ready and just let it happen; I trust them, but damn! It is one weird sensation.

Still no date on the radiation. She (the radiation master) was waiting for Driscoll's e-mail. I will likely see her at the end of this coming week, and then we'll talk about when to start, likely in the last week of February. I stopped to see the radiation nurse Thursday afternoon, and we spoke about timing, etc. My only agenda is to be finished by April vacation, and I should be able to accomplish this without compromising treatment. I will see Driscoll upon his return from vacation on the twenty-fifth when he will inject more saline into the expander.

I'm glad I am doing this, but again, what a concept.

I am growing gradually used to the sight of Dolly's new look. My first glimpse, at my first visit with Driscoll, was enough to have me sobbing later in the morning. That was last week, the day Duke took off. I have since been applying hydrogen peroxide, and have been taking brief showers, so little by little I am letting it sink in. I have to say that since the pathology report, my attitude has changed somewhat. I am grateful that although it meant the complete sacrifice of Dolly, it was not in vain, and whatever the look, it is the look of life. When I am able to just be curious and amazed by science and technology, I can be fascinated by the changes that Dolly will continue to undergo in the next weeks and months. In the meantime, a lot of deep breathing when I need it will help.

And now for the hard part. On Thursday morning, Fran was kind enough to make the very difficult call to me as I was on my way in to see Resciniti, my surgeon. She did not want me to hear on the news that our colleague Diruhi, who uses the office next door to mine, was murdered in the home of a client while doing a home visit. The 18-year-old who took Diruhi's life attempted to take his own, but was alive when found and taken to the hospital (Diruhi had been able to call 911.) I am looking forward to returning to work, and need very much to see my other colleagues and friends there. I'm anticipating a heaviness there that may take some time to work through, and I am hoping that I have the emotional stamina necessary.

I walked into Resciniti's office as I hung up the phone and burst into tears. This was not my usual M.O., and the staff was startled and concerned. When I explained the reason for my tears, one of them said she had heard the news that morning so she knew what I was just learning.

Diruhi had been on my Breasty Business distribution list, asking to be placed there because she had been through this several years ago. She was a frequent responder, offering encouragement, a smile, and in the beginning, when she did not understand my sense of humor, would ask for clarifying information. She would sound confused about something until I could reassure her that I had been joking, teasing. Later she remarked that she was enjoying my "figurative writing." She became concerned when I wrote about having rats and wasn't sure whether I meant that we had rats at home or at the office. She was relieved that in this case I was not writing figuratively, but was being more literal, and that the rats we had named were invited guests who lived in a cage.

The question from her that left me the most stunned was "Do you always have this much fun, or is it just since having treatment?" WHAT??! More fun now? NO, No, No, No! I stopped and remembered that we were just getting to know each other. She would be unaware of how I choose to live my life, the so called humor that I inflict on others, and the importance for me to live my life *even though* I am having treatment. She seemed to see her role as one of mentor, since she had been through treatment herself, although I was not seeking this. I will miss her good intentions.

February 10, 2008
Spice Girl

This would be a reference to my downy crop of salt and pepper hair that is starting to populate my dome. Tiny bits of it may start showing beneath my wig, but there is no way in hell that I will snip these little wisps. You would probably need your microscope to even notice, but if I am to notice all the other odd bits, I should at least get to notice the new fur, eh what?

Gale and I saw Alvin Ailey this afternoon (I think they should join forces with the Chipmunks, don't you?). They were professional, amazing dancers. I think I was more wowed, though, by the choreography of Paul Taylor last fall, as Taylor was more innovative. Ailey is on the traditional side of Modern Dance, but strong and gorgeous. How's that for snobby? It was a lovely outing, and I threatened to do a wig removal only one time.

I am still in search of the perfect bra. Duke accompanied me yesterday to the lingerie department of Kohl's where we took home at least eight to try. There are a couple that will be fine when I am less tender, but for now I'm stuck with the corset job, which is just a tad over the top. Actually, it fastens in the front, so it doesn't have to be over the top. It's okay, but by the time I find the right thing, I will probably not need it anymore. For some reason it irks me to have to put energy into this.

Duke was a saint as I had my trying-on session. It produced fresh tears for me; I didn't want to put him through the adjustment of dealing with my changed self. Despite his reassurances that it was not an issue, I still felt bad, and had to slog my way through. It must have been a useful exercise, though, because I feel better now. Maybe it was just being able to share that with him that I needed. Logic does not always rule the day, and I don't always need to understand *why* something is, just that it is.

February 12, 2008
Hi ho, hi ho....

It's off to work I go. Despite the intense sadness surrounding the loss of Diruhi, I was very excited to get to work yesterday and today. I enjoy the work that I do, but it has been a long time since I felt that level of excitement about going in. It was good to have the energy and focus to devote to it, and it was really important to see my work mates. My colleagues have responded amazingly well to this tragic event, dedicating themselves to the young adult daughters of Diruhi and sorting through the complicated web of confidentiality around her clients.

Among us, we will be represented at both the wake and funeral this week. It has been very dense going, and I know that there are many layers still to come, but I'm glad that I have, at least, returned to some semblance of life as I know it. A visit with the radiation oncologist tomorrow will bring more information about that process.

More soon…oh bla di oh bla da life goes on…bra!

February 13, 2008
Put Off

So I saw my Laser Lady today and was unfortunately not able to complete the planning session. The radiology technicians need to do a session with my arms up over my head, and my surgical arm is not able to do this yet. I had been specifically not using it too much because of Driscoll voicing his concern about popping an internal stitch. This is probably the only downside to having two surgeons at once. They each were deferring to the other in terms of activity level, and so I did not get a lot of clear direction. Had I known what was involved in the planning session, I would have made sure to be stretching more than I have. Anyway, I am rescheduled for the planning session on Leap Day, with radiation to begin the first week in March. I don't have an exact date yet, but I will call and ask for this in my attempt to stay ahead of the game in terms of scheduling for work. Hugs was right about the six week time frame to wait post surgery before beginning with the heat

I am excited about Leap Day, especially as it occurs on a Friday and seems even more celebratory than it normally would. A time to move forward, to do something one might not normally do. This year that includes for me an appointment with Hugs in the morning, and an appointment with the Radiant One in the afternoon.

She was talking to me about possible complications today, and when she came to arm edema, I smiled. She looked quizzical, so I admitted that every time she says that, I hear armadillo, and I smile to think of these curious creatures. She said that she hadn't heard that one and wanted to add it to some list she has. Anyway, I am disappointed not to be getting going (and finished) with Triathlon Phase III, but I know that we are on our way, and probably starting only a week later than I thought. This is where I have to remind myself that in the big scheme of things, it is really nothing at all. Patience, as I have said, is a challenge.

What a snow/rain day we are having!!!

February 17, 2008
Walking the Walk

This is a literal one. On Friday, when the mercury topped 40 degrees, I took to the streets. First Kate and I walked to greet her arriving friends, and since this was way too short, I did my 3-mile loop up the hill. It was wonderful to be outside, and moving around a little. I was admittedly a wee tad tired Friday night, but it felt great.

I took a little field trip to the boob store, as my friend Dodie named it. The Women's Image Center is a terrific resource. I had been there when I was researching reconstruction options, and it is through this place that I learned about external reconstruction. It is a one-person-at-a-time operation (bad pun) and feels very personal. Mary, the owner, took more than our half hour allotted slot, and found just the right shaped bra without underwire that works perfectly for me. She even threw in a bra expander (this does not expand the entire bra, like a balloon, which is what I pictured when she mentioned it—it just adds a couple of hooks onto the end so that when you need it to be a little looser, it can be. This will be especially key during radiation, because chafing is apparently one of the biggest issues during this time). I was thrilled with the visit, because just three weeks after surgery, I can wear one of these bras and look pretty normal, or at least wear normalish clothes.

She was impressed with my reconstruction, as I am not that far off from where I started. The whole thing is pretty amazing. Best yet, it's all covered under insurance! This visit could be an essay in itself, but I will desist for the moment.

I took a minor spill on the ice today, and feel a little sore, but it could have been a whole lot worse. I am working my arm, slowly, and am getting greater range of motion daily. It is a discipline, but I have a very specific target, which helps.

In the end, I'm glad for the time to heal before radiation. The stronger I go in, the easier it will be. I feel pretty good, but am still not 100 percent, obviously. I do have energy, but I'm trying to be careful about how I use it, as it is not boundless at the moment.

Duke and I had an unexpected date when both Gale and Kate were out for the night! So nice. There is never enough time for each other, or with those girls.

February 24, 2008
Lull a Bye Bye

This past week was the lull with no appointments, the (relative) calm before the maelstrom of appointments starting this week. I have four, and radiation doesn't start until next week sometime. It has been a curious week, a mix of emotions and physical sensations.

Physically, I feel strong, and have a fair amount of energy, enough so that it was a relief to go for my walk yesterday and today in the bright, cold sunshine. It has been beautiful, with all the fresh snow draped over tree and lawn.

My surgical site is still sore, and I have been having trouble sorting out the bra scene. I think it is the reconstruction that makes me tender so that the bra feels like it is digging in still. My skin is sensitive in general in the whole area, sometimes making it difficult to have anything at all against it. I briefly considered renaming Dolly and Parton as Mutt and Jeff but that seems rude.

I know this will get better, but in the meantime it's a bit of a challenge figuring out how to be comfortable and symmetrical. Some people will tell you that symmetry is overrated, but I'm here to tell you that it has its place. Anyway, without going into greater detail, suffice to say that where some people change their clothes many times a day, I am adjusting my bra-ness to suit. It's so odd. And a bit tiring.

I'm slowly starting to show off my up-and-coming do. Still not ready to abandon the Critter and many hats completely, but hopefully by spring, when it's warmed up a bit, I will also be ready to debut the new look. It has crossed my mind to have my ears pierced. I mentioned this thought to Duke, who could barely contain his enthusiasm ("Think of the gift possibilities!"). He thinks I'm toying with him. I probably should have kept my mouth shut, as I am nowhere near convinced that I want to do this.

"It's fun!" Gale has encouraged me.

I know she's right, but the momentum has still not gathered in this direction, and so for now I will continue to direct my jewelry energy to my neck and wrist, and see what happens as I get closer to doffing my wig. Am I ready for so much change at once? That is part of it. If I thought the wig provoked reactions, I'm sure that the removal of it will provoke more (unless people are just shocked into silence). I love to wave my head about in its fuzzy freedom anyway, so it doesn't matter. My family, and friends Pam and Phil, are all encouraging the natural look.

Earlier in the week, I was feeling mad about Diruhi's tragic death, angry not only that it had happened, but in my selfishness, angry that my workplace had been covered with grief. It was one place that had not been so affected by all that has been happening. I was not ready to gather with people about it. As the week went on, however, my energy seeped back in, and I was looking forward to being with my colleagues and gathering in a group, which we do not often do. The snow intervened, and I did not drive up for the evening event, but I know now that we will get together another time, and that our sense of being a group of sorts is cemented in a way that it never has been before. Diruhi would be pleased about this.

BIG NEWS! Gale was accepted at Goucher College! There's even a possibility of some scholarship money pending the receipt of her mid-year "grades." Yea! I'm thrilled for her, but then it hit me this afternoon—she's really going to college next year. Even if it's not there, at Goucher, it somehow began to sink in that this is for real. Hey, how did that sneak up like that? Yikes!!!

Well, tomorrow starts new adventures in medical land with another visit to Plastsic Guy. I've also re-contacted Mr. Magic, of acupuncture fame, to address both post-surgical issues and radiation effects. If I'm experiencing "breakthrough heat" now, I can just imagine what will happen with radiation. Who knows what I'll be breaking through? The sound barrier? The boiling point? We'll find out. Hope you all had a chance to get out and enjoy the sunshine.

February 24, 2008
Lancealittle....

Lance Armstrong is, by anyone's definition, one of the most tenacious, astoundingly single-minded and determined people on the planet. His single-mindedness when it came to addressing his illness or the Tour de France was nothing short of astonishing. I was fascinated to read about both the political and strategic aspects of the tour, to say nothing of the physical stamina he developed. His physique changed after his illness, making him a bit more streamlined, better designed for endurance than for sprinting, which had previously been his specialty.

His illness was so different from what I have encountered that it can hardly be said to dwell under the same umbrella (and this not even a rainy day…). What he endured was more intense in every dimension—his treatment rendered him far sicker, and his disease was far more acute and aggressive. He had to take time off from what he had been doing, and it redefined his life in a dramatic way.

I have been able to continue with my life in almost all aspects, and perhaps I have been tenacious about this. I know what I want to continue to do and what I want to start doing when my treatment ends, and my lessons have been different (more about this another time).

Armstrong defines courage as "the quality of spirit that enables one to encounter danger with firmness and without fear." I believe it involves being able to act and continue even in the face of fear. Sometimes having courage means not only allowing the fear to enter, but asking for help in dealing with it. It takes courage to be vulnerable. They are not mutually exclusive properties. I don't even know how I would describe danger. Ana once told me that I calculate out the risks involved in doing something so that I do not see them as risks. Again, I had not really considered this; I suppose this is true, because once I see where I want to go, it is really a matter of getting the stepping stones into place, whatever that means, in a given situation. And then it is not so much about risks, as figuring out how to put each stone into place with as much clarity as I can breathe into it.

Whew! Just had to get that out. Sometimes when I don't write for a while (like 3½ minutes), stuff crowds in there demanding an exit, and who am I to get in the way? It'll just take up space and distract me until I download it, and thank you for being there with your catcher's mitts to receive all these thoughts. It's much more satisfying than mumbling to myself, which is apparently already a specialty of mine.

Okay, I'm signing off for the moment, but no promises about not returning soon.

February 27, 2008
Frogs at the ready

So are you all preparing for LEAP DAY? It is this Friday, you know. The perfect time to try something new, say something you've been meaning to say, try a new food. Or just jump a lot. Or leap about with your doctors, because I can't think of anything more fun than that. Do you think I can get them to leap, because you know I'm going to bring up this leaping business. There will be times when I will need to be very still, but in between, bring on the frogs, baby.

And by the way, I saw Plastic Guy on Monday. He filled the tissue expander to where it needs to be, which means that my skin is taut and kind of uncomfortable. He found the port to fill it by using a magnet (isn't that cool?), and then attached a syringe to a bag of saline solution and injected it. The whole thing took less than 10 minutes, with me babbling and trying not to watch too closely. He had been out with a hernia operation and was feeling a little uncomfortable himself, and said that he has more sympathy than he had before for post-surgical discomfort.

He asked about the radiation, and I told him it has been delayed because I couldn't do the planning session. He didn't know that I would need to have my arms up above my head for 45 minutes in order to do this. Of course I wouldn't be able to do it 2½ weeks post-op.

Interesting.

I don't think she (Laser Lady) realized that my range of motion so soon after mastectomy and reconstruction would be what it is. Driscoll pointed out that radiation typically follows chemotherapy, so that it would be several months past the surgery itself. Or, if it is a simple lumpectomy without lymph node removal, range of motion would not be so affected.

There needs to be some more education among the docs, I think. They *are* communicating; they're just missing some of how their various services interact with each other. Or maybe I'm underestimating the newness of how I'm going about this. It's a little hard for me to tell. I don't want to compromise my recovery in any way, so I'm paying close attention to each doc and asking questions when there seems to be a contradiction or inconsistency in my treatment.

February 27, 2008
Point of Gale Information

I realized that it was confusing about Gale's Goucher acceptance. She applied there early action, but not early decision, so although we are all tickled, she is still waiting to hear from a number of other schools, along with their financial offerings, before making a final decision (sometime in late April). Ye ha!!!

March 2, 2008
Latest Shenanigans

Sometimes it takes me a couple of days to digest what goes down in my appointments, even if they don't seem all that dramatic on the surface. Having two in one day perhaps compounded the experience. However, it was LEAP DAY and I did, in fact, make the wig leap! Done with the wig! Off of my head! The Critter now sits on top of my bureau, awaiting instruction. I noticed that my shampoo, the same bottle I bought last August, is called Fresh Curls. How apt. Once those curls commence, if they commence, they could not be more fresh!

The first place I went on Leap Day was to see Hugs, whose office staff is totally accustomed to seeing people in very short hair, wigs, and every manner of hat, kerchief, or head topping. No one blinked an eye (and you should see them with all their eyes needing to blink). Hugs was the only one who commented outright, although he said that he did like my wig. He also assumed that I was not happy about my hair, for some reason. He made some allusion to perfectionism, but he is wrong about my feelings about my hair. I'm thrilled that it's making a return, and although of course I want it to please hurry up, I'm happy to see it coming back at all.

Hugs reminded me that what they expect after surgery is for people to be breathing, all their parts working, and able to feed themselves. After that it's all gravy (Yuck). It was a good reminder for me not to take how I feel, or my recovery, for granted. He asked how much of my energy is back; was it 40 percent, 70 percent, 90 percent? I thought about it for a second and realized that it was probably around 90 percent, although clearly the flexibility in my arm is nowhere near that, and what I'm able to do with it is not near that either. I can do a lot, but anything to do with lifting or opening tough jars is out (arm, you ahr owt; rest of the body, you ahr in!). In any event, I am grateful that I feel as well as I do, despite the fact that it is still completely bizarre to deal with the surgical area, from every standpoint.

Again, he made some reference to expecting perfection, but I don't even know what that is, or what he is talking about. I have very little in the way of a reference point, and so I am not measuring myself against anything, which has worked for me. I am just doing what feels right for me and doing what I can do. Yes, I expect a lot in terms of what I aim for in recovery, but I have no idea what anyone else does, or how quickly or slowly, and it doesn't matter anyway. I am not in competition with anyone, nor do I have exact time frames in mind for when I can do what. I do expect to bike this spring and swim this summer, and I think that's reasonable. I would love to ski again this winter, but that may not happen, although with the amount of snow we keep getting, it will likely be possible in Vermont deep into the spring!

Hugs was delighted by the pathology report, which took me by surprise. He said that with multifocal cancer going into surgery, it was possible to expect to find more and larger spots in the pathology, and the fact that there was only one, and that it was measured in millimeters, was a terrific result. That it was close to the margin does not at all concern him, particularly as I will be starting radiation therapy.

He talked again about Tamoxifen, the oral therapy to begin some-time in the next several weeks. I balked a little, just because it was another thing. He has mentioned it before and given me literature, but my usual multitasking self is really taking this treatment thing one step at a time, and I just had not thought about it much. I'm concerned about the side effects, but he assured me that I am not at high risk for any of them, and should not be so worried, because many women do not expe-rience any. It may augment any menopausal symptoms. He noted again that some women do restart their cycle, even a year after chemotherapy, so I should be aware of this vis-a-vis birth control. I assured him that my husband was not about to reverse his vasectomy. He just looked down and shook his head a little. The Tamoxifen is the best preventive measure so once I get around to focusing on this, I'll be grateful for its protection.

Ana and I walked and ate before my next appointment. I had to pick one of the coldest days for my wiggie freedom. Good thing I have such cute fleece hats to choose from.

The radiology technicians and my radiation oncologist were pleased that my increased mobility allowed me to complete the planning session for radiotherapy (yes, radios need therapy, too). It was not hard to do. It was, as Laser Lady suggested, a matter of how I focus my attention. I needed a little pad under my arm, and then she (Lena) taped it in place for the CT scan and the marking session. Lena got me into the position needed, and then I had to lie still about five minutes or so for the CT scan. Next, while Dr. Schoenthaler did the computations, Lena took my arms down, but I had to continue to lie still, including my head and legs, for another 10 – 15 minutes. For the marking session, she reposed my arms, and then first marked five spots with a sharpie, then came back and marked each spot using a needle and India ink. These are tiny little pricks (still talking about the needle here), but it killed any thoughts I had about going to the ear piercing pagoda afterward.

It took a lot of focus for me to lie that still for all that time. It also took some luck; I only had one bout of severely needing to scratch my nose. Thankfully, Lena figured out that if she talked to me from behind my head I would be tempted to turn and look at her, so she came over to the other side.

None of it was all that traumatic, but it still took awhile. Just to make things more time-consuming, I had a session with the nurse to tell me about skin care, during which she noticed that the hospital gown I happened to choose was ripped to the point where she asked to get me a new one for her sake. (Sweet that she was embarrassed by the office's tatty gowns.) The biggest issues are the burning and the skin sensitivity, so she gave me a gel to use twice a day. She also told me to get cornstarch to apply liberally and frequently to cut down on the friction. I will certainly heed this advice, as my skin is still sensitive from the surgery. Then she sent me on yet another bra-shopping extravaganza. I stopped on the way home and picked up a stretchy, all-cotton job with a wide band on the bottom, which seems good.

None of them are perfect, and they all drive me crazy after a few hours, but in different ways. So maybe if I switch them up I can at least have some variety in my loonyness. And it is better. Definitely less sensitive this week.

They also needed to take another picture of me for my photo ID, because Lena (who had not been there during my visit 2½ weeks ago) didn't recognize me without the wig at first. I got a parking pass so that I can pull into the special lot and not have to pay for parking. I also don't have to check in at the front desk; I can go right to the back, get changed and ready for radio fun. They really are trying to streamline this thing so that, even though it's every day, there is that much less hassle.

I appreciate this, because it all makes a difference. Starting Thursday, I will be greeting them on a daily basis at 8 a.m.

That's the long and short of it. On Friday night, Duke and I went with Kate to the Bull Run to see one of her friends play in a band, and that was my first major public time without the Critter. I didn't catch anyone sniggering, so I took this to be a good sign. It is freeing, and I do like it when people pat my fuzzy head. There's a side of me that's part pooch.

Gale and I are doing a flying Goucher visit, arriving Tuesday eve, and returning Wednesday. Purchase College invited her (by e-mail) to an accepted students day, so we assumed that meant she was, in fact, accepted. This was confirmed by post two days later. And now we wait for the rest until April.

March 2, 2008
In praise of eyebrows

The eyebrows were the last to go, and as they're coming in, they don't have to grow very much. That's a good thing. I still need some filler, but less.

I was thinking about the marking session and remembered that when I was waiting, in between the CT scan and the marking, Lena gave me a firm foam donut to hold in order to keep still. Also, she taped my arm when it was up to keep it still. These are meant to be helpful things, and they are, but they also both add to the seriousness of the whole thing, and the intensity of the experience. They do not want to take the risk of any movement, so they gently imprison people's limbs. It's draining.

No concentration right now for any more.

Chapter 4

Taking the Heat

March 6, 2008
Radiotherapy

I figured out why the radios need therapy. It's another hair issue. Do they want long waves or short....

March 6, 2008
Boulder

This would be referring to what was on my chest when I left my appointment on Monday afternoon with the Plastic Guy. I had gone to the appointment expecting it to be for a brief check, "oh, very nice; everything's fine" and then be on my way. I had met Susan for a quick walk beforehand, and even invited her to wait for me because I thought we would have time to walk more afterward, given the brevity of my appointment.

This was not to be.

What had I missed? My understanding was that he wanted to fill the tissue expander once more before starting radiation. That was last week, and we had thought I would already be starting radiation this week.

Evidently, he wanted to fill it more, and asked what Laser Lady thought. I had not even brought it up this time because I thought it was not going to happen; that I was done. So we talked about it for a bit, and I remembered that she said that filling it shouldn't change the pattern that was already tattooed, that it should expand up, not out, kind of like adding more rings to the center of a topographic map. We went around for a bit, and finally decided to go ahead.

He used a small needle at first, and after a few minutes became impatient with the slow rate of fill, so he asked the nurse for a larger one. The first needle had barely hurt at all, but the second one was a jab that made me jump. That combined with the more rapid fill rate, which stretched my skin much more quickly, left me feeling unprepared, and like someone was standing on my chest. The quease factor began to kick in, and I asked for some water. The nurse went to get it for me. He stopped 20 ml short of the 100 ml he wanted to add, and told me to make another appointment in a couple of weeks. The nurse could see that I was a bit off balance, and told me to take my time getting out of the room. Partly it was the expectations thing, and partly it was just that this procedure can be uncomfortable, and I had not been ready.

I was a bit teary-eyed following this episode, and really uncomfortable. The nurse reminded me that this works kind of like getting braces; the physical adjustment is uncomfortable for a few days until the skin adapts. In the meantime, it's a little hard to breathe, bringing new meaning to the term "over the shoulder boulder holder." I was too uncomfortable to go to my group, and Susan took me to Starbuck's for water to wash down some Tylenol before I headed home to crack something stronger, like a Wachusett Ale.

Today is Day 1 of Radiation. I hope my arm is up to the task.

Gale and I had a good trip to Goucher. Our flight down was delayed by two hours because of weather and a crew change, but was otherwise uneventful. Goucher is pretty and interesting, and it remains a contender. We didn't really learn anything new, except that it will be fine if Gale ends up here. She'll wait to hear from the rest of the schools before making a decision next month. It was nice to have a little time out-of-time, and we were able to do a little prom dress shopping while we waited to go out to the airport for our return flight. Although entertaining, the shopping was in vain, which is not a good place to look for dresses.

On to my next escapade.

March 6, 2008
Kickin' Some Radiation Butt

I got to use my little wand (aka credit card like thing that I wave in front of the parking lot arm) to get into the primo lot at Emerson. I waltzed past the reception desk and pulled out a robe that had two ties, got into it, and a few minutes later was ushered into the room with the radiation thing happening. They took x-rays to verify that my position on the radiation table lined up with where they had me set-up initially. Next they irradiated three places on my chest, and sent me back out into the sun washed morning without stopping to check out/pay co-pays, etc. They commented on how well I'm doing with my arm. Maybe they won't use tape next time.

I was given a gel to use on my entire upper left quadrant to help keep it supple (starting now) and told to use copious amounts of corn-starch once my skin becomes sensitive. They're worried about friction (and we're not talking Pulp Friction) being the main offender as radiation goes on. I will probably look like a powdered puff pastry by the end of the day once I start with that stuff.

In the meantime, this thing will be very do-able. All the little steps that are saved count: I appreciate economy of motion. It will get old to drive there every day, so it's nice that this is a short week, and that tomorrow I don't have to go rushing off to work right after.

I'm officially launched on the third leg of my Triathlon! Yea!! Is it possible that there really is an end to this thing?

March 7, 2008
Diagnostic Tool

This is what we in the Biz refer to when evaluating clients sometimes. If you ask the same question in the same way to many different people, you learn something about each of them when you get the answer. In my old office, I had a plant (literally) that was like a diagnostic tool. The office was very large and rectangular shaped. The entrance was at one end of the rectangle, and I had a large plant (named Fred) that took up a lot of the back part of the space. The seating area, desk, etc., were at the other end. The plant had large leaves, and it had air roots that snaked around the office. Often, the leaves would hang over the edge of the couch, and just about tap someone sitting there on the shoulder. Sometimes, after seeing a client for six months, he would come in and say, "Hey, you got a new plant!" I knew that a person was feeling better if he or she had started to notice Fred.

Some clients advised me on how to care for Fred. He needed repotting, he needed the air roots trimmed, or not trimmed, or whatever. Certainly almost anyone knows more than I do about plants, so I know that some of this was good advice. That I managed to keep Fred alive is remarkable in itself, but it was fascinating to see who noticed it, who didn't, and who commented. Not a perfect tool, but interesting.

My wig removal has similarly sparked some interesting responses, and teaches me about my clients (although sometimes a wig is just a wig...). The very first client who I saw after leaving the wig at home, is herself five years past her own breast cancer diagnosis, and has gone through the whole boat of treatment. She loved the non-wig look, and was very complimentary about how she thought it was strong and chic looking. It totally blew her away. She herself never wore her wig because it freaked her daughter out and was also uncomfortable to wear. The next client noted that it was different, but observed, "It looks good," and she was on to something else. A couple of clients said absolutely nothing at all. I'm not sure whether they were taken aback, or didn't know what to say, or in one case, I'm pretty sure that what was going on in the client's life was more than enough to deal with. There was not time to discuss my new coif.

Newer clients who are unaware of my treatment took note, and I had thought I would need to explain, but in fact that was not necessary. People do sometimes radically change their hairstyles. They have no idea that this is not something I usually do.

When I went to meet my last client of the day yesterday, I looked down the long corridor, and thought I saw her in the doorway of the waiting room. I looked a little more closely, and then started walking down toward her. It was starting to get dark, so the light was a little odd. She stood up and started walking toward me.

"I wasn't quite sure that was you," I said to her. "Your hair looks a little different." We both laughed as we realized the irony of what I had just said. "I guess not as different as my hair looks," I added.

Earlier in the day, I greeted the man in the office next door, asked how he was doing. He shared the office with Diruhi, and I know he had known her a long time.

"I don't think we've met," he said.

I introduced myself (again), and I realized much later that he probably didn't recognize me without the wig! I had become enough accustomed to it that I almost forgot how radically different it looks.

Anyway, it is amusing. We'll see what next week's sessions bring... maybe I'll try to get a photo out so that you, too, can tell me whether I do in fact look like a snowy owl. Gale says no, that my head doesn't turn all the way around. Good thing, because that is an Exorcist trick I would rather not bring to mind.

Time for Mr. Dog's constitutional...he'll be pleased.

March 11, 2008
Having Your Head Eggsamined....

The Church Board in Ayer often has head-scratching kinds of homilies displayed as we drive past on our way to Parker, the girls' school, or Kate's gymnastics. The past (rather mundane) one had been there an unusually long time, but when we rode past yesterday I noticed that it was offering new and different thoughts. The comment this time is, "No bunny has ever died for you."

Clearly, I am aware of this.

My mind went immediately to thinking that there was some word play about no **body** instead of bunny. "What?!" I cried. Kate submitted that they're suggesting that people focus too much on the Easter Bunny, who has not, in fact, sacrificed himself for us. I'm sure that she's right, and I then was searching for some other image than a giant bunny on a cross.

As I groped for an alternative, Kate said, "All I can imagine is Jesus going from house to house with all those Easter baskets." Ah, that was much more comforting. Hopefully he's tiptoeing through the tulips as he goes....

Radiation continues uneventfully. My daily time gets moved up to 7:50 tomorrow morning, which will make it less stressful to get to work in Andover at 9:00 on Mondays and Tuesdays. It's weird that this painless procedure is so powerful. I'm hoping that as my skin gets less sensitive from the surgery it does not immediately become more sensitive from the rads. And to think: all this has less impact than the hormone therapy to start soon. It's amazing.

Hair reactions continue.

One client, who'd seen the new hair last Monday, said "There's twice as much," in her matter-of-fact way, then went on to other things.

Another client today mentioned that her hair is the only part of her that she has always loved, and that she never wanted to mess with it in any way. Seeing my patchy fuzz (my words, not hers), she remarked that it inspired her to see it so radically different, and yet to still like it.

Hope you are enjoying the day. It's sunny and brisk here, and I managed to get out in it for a little while. I'm starting to get that cycling itch.

March 12, 2008
Graze Anatomy

This is what happens when you eat all day long. I suppose that cows must be quite expert.

I meet weekly with my Laser Lady as I move through this phase of the triathlon. She had told me earlier that it would depend on my exact anatomy how much involvement my heart and lungs would have. Hopefully, not too much. I met with her today and asked her about this. She showed me an amazing cross-section printout with color-coded beams on it. A tiny part of what she does is to work out the best route for the beams while minimizing other organ involvement. "Almost none at all," is how much my heart and lungs will be hit. So my heart is in the right place after all.

"You have excellent anatomy," she joked. Again, I'll take it. I don't care how little I had to do with it (although she did say that athletes' lungs tend to lie flatter). It's a tiny thing, but it made me smile.

I also need to get on the cornstarch thing. I'm not supposed to wait for the skin tenderness; the idea is to be cutting down on friction Now. So I'll start poofing away, and I can take a day off from radiation here or there if I want to accompany Gale to an "accepted students day." I will just need to tack the day on to the end of the treatment.

So there we are.

March 14, 2008
Philosophical Question

What did Aristotle wear to football matches? Think…no groaning aloud….

Soccertees! Who else, but?

March 14, 2008
Hair Today….

I learned today that following 28 treatments of the type I am receiving now, I will have potentially from 5 – 7 "booster" rads of a different, electron-based type, to a different area, namely the scar area from the excision of the original lump. The technician I saw today didn't know if, or how many, as the script hadn't been written yet. I will ask Laser Lady when I see her next Wednesday. I'm not sure how the set of criteria for this is determined. We'll see.

I am also trying to be compliant with the Natural Care Gel/cornstarch regimen, although thus far I am failing. The gel takes a while to dry, which is an issue when I'm struggling to get my ass out the door in the morning, or into PJs at night. And I am forgetting the cornstarch. Duke did put some in an adorable little talcum powder container, so that will help with the mess issue. Maybe I need to put it into some funky little dog or cat salt shaker so that it will make me smile each time I go to use it.

I am caught between the experience of the radiation oncology nurses across many patients, and my knowledge of my own body. Plus, at this stage there is no discomfort, so there is not a bodily reminder (I know, Noah was building his ark without the aid of weather people…). And the camisole is okay, but not ideal. I may need to mix up my undergarments so that I'm not wearing any one thing too often (okay, I'll continue to make the panties a regular thing…). I have to have some trust that I am doing what I can to minimize friction, even if that does mean wearing a regular bra sometimes. With the extenders, it really can be pretty loose while still doing its designated job. I'm pretty sure that this is a comfort issue, not safety, and that if I don't follow strictly to the letter that I'm not screwing up my ultimate care. My stillness on the table is more vital. And showing up for treatment.

I had my first comment from a complete stranger today. About my hair, that is. I was wandering about Trader Joe's loading my cart with every imaginable snack item (why did I go there when I was hungry?) when a fellow shopper said to me, "I love your hair!"

I turned to face a woman probably 10 years younger with short dark hair. She continued, "I usually wear mine like that, too. I'm just growing it out right now."

I recovered from my cookie reverie to say "Thank you. It's different for me, but it's fun."

"Has anyone called you sir, yet?" she asked. WHAT? This had not occurred to me. Just never know where my imagination will fall short.

"No, not yet," I told her. Something to look forward to though, eh?

"Well, it looks good," she said, and wheeled her cart away. Had I forgotten to take down my "Please tell me about my hair" nametag? I continue to marvel at the unexpected turns this journey will take.

The best part, though, is the richness that has developed in so many relationships, family and friends alike. I continue to be grateful for the depth and breadth of what you bring to this lengthy and circuitous chapter in my life.

Enjoy the weekend. Spring really is coming.

March 18, 2008
Corn Starch Kid

First of all, before I forget, you must know that one of the most fascinating substances ever is oobleck. It is one of the few uses for corn-starch I have come across apart from my present one. If you have not created this magical, multi-propertied stuff while in preschool, or with preschoolers, you must treat yourself. It is simply cornstarch and water, and it can pour like a viscous liquid and be contained like a solid. So it oozes, and slimes, and also adheres to itself. It simply must be in your repertoire if you are under, say, 100 years old.

That said, I went to CVS today to expand my repertoire of cornstarch-administering tools. Roe and I discussed powder puffs. I asked the nice young goateed man where I might find one of these. I expected him to look for my second head, which must surely be lolling about somewhere, and then tell me that I can find them out back in the Model-T Ford, but he marched straight to the makeup area and waved a hand at the array of brushes that are used to apply foundation, blush, etc.

I had several to choose from (Stand Up, purse, Kabuki, and Kabuki retractable, along with those more specifically for blush, shadow, etc.). I chose one Stand Up (as in either comedic, or dependable) to hang out on my dresser, and one Kabuki retractable to travel with me. I have tried out the Stand Up, and I must say that there is simply no way to do this neatly. It does absolutely help, better than just dumping the box down my shirt. I'm going to end up like Pig Pen's counterpart. While he traveled about in a black cloud of dirt, I will travel in a haze of white. It's going to make me think of all the pastries that are dusted with powdered sugar, but it is disappointingly about as delightful as unsweetened chocolate.

All this to create a new habit. I'm trying not to whine and make excuses. I believe that it is no coincidence when our clients mirror our own issues, and so it should be no surprise that two clients, after I have been meeting with them for months, have chosen now to deal with breaking old habits, namely smoking and overeating. They each need to create new habits, and make this a priority in order to make it work. I, too, must do this, and I don't have a ton of time in which to do it. I do not have the luxury of considering it, rolling it around in my mouth for awhile as I decide how to proceed. I need to get on the Corn Starch Train right away. And so I am trying to be jiggy with it, welcome it, and get it in place.

It seems absurd, all this focus on Corn Starch, but it is temporary.

I have had more feedback. Yesterday's input was from a co-worker who I don't see very often, as he is usually only in the office on Tuesday evenings, and I leave by two or three. He didn't recognize me at first, but responded when I said hello, and we had a minute to chat. He asked how things are going and offered to be available should I need someone to talk with. I assured him that I was talking (and have 80 people who can attest to that) and really feel like I'm getting a lot out. I started trotting downstairs, and he said that I have changed.

I stopped mid-stair (and mid-stare) and asked, "My hair?"

"No," he replied. "Your personality." Uh-oh.

I might have raced down the rest of the stairs, but I had to know. "How so?"

"You're more self-assured," he told me. Well, I'll be damned!

Duke roared with laughter when he heard this. "Oh yes, you've finally shed that timid, retiring part of yourself." But I find it interesting, and it is my vow to honor what is offered to me in a positive way. Maybe there is something different in the way I am presenting myself. Hmmmmmm.

I have met with more clients who are seeing the change for the first time. One of them is a client who I have known for years. She was in treatment (counseling) for probably around a year the first time, maybe 15 years ago. Then she was back for a few sessions six or seven years ago. I went out to the waiting room to greet her.

"Hey!" I called.

"It's been years!" she called back. She looked up at me and paused. I could see her mind sorting files. This is not what she was expecting. Finally, she declared "You look fabulous!"

I have been so used to looking the same, I hadn't realized quite how vested in this I have been until I suddenly looked very different. Some people do this by choice, and frequently. I have kept my hair largely the same for years (with the aid of chemicals). My dress has changed somewhat, but not hugely. My weight has been roughly the same (without the aid of chemicals). So, it is just an unaccustomed thing to have such a dramatic change, and to hear about it. I was ready, and I must say, it has been absolutely fascinating, and fortunately mostly positive (the naysayers being too polite to shout it out).

It is part of my lesson, somehow, all this focus on my appearance. I wouldn't go on about it so, except somehow it is highlighting that the inside is in many ways exactly the same, and in others can't possibly be. There is something trying to surface about balance and what is important, and it being okay to put myself out there, but there has been too much day in my day to make more sense of it right now. I'll be back when it surfaces.

Tomorrow I visit with the Corn Starch Patrol. I'll let you know how it goes.

March 19, 2008
28

This is the total number of radiation sessions that I will receive, 10 of which I have already completed, which means that I am more than a third of the way through! Sometimes they do the boosters of 5 – 7 sessions, but not in my case because of the type of surgery. So, I'm looking at finishing those sometime in the middle of April, depending on whether I end up taking days off for any reason.

Still no reaction to the radiation, which is what they expect. I did learn that sometimes people's skin breaks down, necessitating time off from the radiation and thereby extending the total time. This happens most often in cases in which there is a lot of friction and/or moisture that contributes to the condition. The underside of the breast for larger-breasted women is a vulnerable area. My reconstruction has helped to eliminate this issue. Perky girls create less friction. And I'm hoping that my acupuncture is helping to get rid of excess heat in my body, thereby again hopefully helping out the irradiated area.

I need to make a return trip to CVS to look for the powder puff (now it's just a matter of curiosity). Gale's friend Anne suggested that it might be in the body powder section, and that I may need to buy the powder in order to get the Puff. I'll also search out someone a little more matronly to assist in this endeavor, should my own search prove fruitless (and am I really looking for fruit here?).

I see Plastic Guy on Friday, Acupuncture Guy next week, Hugs the week after, so I'm still fairly appointment-dense these next few weeks. I'm hoping it will slow down after the rads are done, at least until we get close to the surgery that swaps the tissue expander for the implant. I don't want to get ahead of myself, though. We'll see how much fluid Driscoll wants to add, and whether there will be more sessions.

Wet weather, low-key day, which is fine.

The cat and the rat are trying to interact with each other, which is interesting. Tobin is climbing up inside the cage and poking his nose through to get a better whiff of Bobcat, who is sitting on the bookcase, calmly studying the rat's every move. Once in a while Bobcat gets closer, and occasionally Tobin will poke him in the paw, making Bobcat retreat. Kate is concerned that there is some kind of reverse interest thing going on. She says this sometimes happens, and is dangerous for the rats because they put themselves in harm's way with the cats instead of retreating from them. I'm hoping that there is just the curiosity of proximity, and that they are forging an interspecies communication.

At any rate, happy midweek to ye.

March 21, 2008
Beam On!!!!!!

I figure this must be the way the radiation people greet or leave one another. It's actually one of three signs that light up outside the radiation room. The first two say Entry Permitted and then No Entry and then Beam On. It sounds kind of Space Exploration-oid and has an upbeat feel to it. I like it.

I have the first radiation slot of the day at 7:50 a.m. There is almost always an older gent there who is tackling the puzzle that is on the table. (His time must be sometime not too long after eight.) The first few days I was too into my book to talk much. Yesterday I helped him with the outline of the puzzle. Today there was a new puzzle and we started discussing why the other one was removed.

At 7:45, a lullaby came over the sound system in the waiting area, while something heavy metal came on in the control room. The contrasting music was curious (I found out a year later that the lullaby meant that a baby is born in the hospital). We were chatting about this, and then he said that I must be almost done with my radiation.

"Well, I'll hit the midpoint next week," I said.

He commented that when people are almost finished, their personalities change, because they're relieved to be at the end of the treatment. He himself has six more to go, so maybe it's his personality that's changing.

The technicians commented that someone must have been in the control room at night and changed the station on the radio. It made me a little nervous, because what if they are also changing things on the machinery?!! I do not tend toward paranoia, but we're talking about a procedure in which accuracy is everything. They will shift me literally millimeters on the board to make sure that I am in exactly the right spot. They take x-rays every five or six days for quality control. Anyway, they assured me that the machinery is just fine, and we proceeded uneventfully.

I saw Driscoll (Plastic Guy) this afternoon. He was tied up in surgery for an extra half hour, which they told me as soon as I arrived. I was shown into the exam room, and I eyed the equipment required to do another fill of the expander. He and his nurse, Karen, came in. He is always accompanied by her, probably to make sure there is a woman present while doing exams. She is right around six feet tall, and he is closer to five foot six, so they make an interesting pair. Yin and Yang in a number of ways. They took a look, we talked for a couple of minutes, and he decided to do…nothing. He is concerned that trying to expand more right now while there is still a few weeks of radiation to go could cause me pain, so we'll leave it as it is.

At first I was disappointed that we didn't proceed as planned, but it is what it is, and Driscoll is using his best judgment with an unusual situation, and I will just keep hoping for the best result. He wants to wait several months after radiation to give the skin time to settle and relax so that there won't be a tendency to tighten up and be painful (or reject the implant altogether).

Anyway, to all of you I say, "Have a good weekend, and BEAM ON!!!"

March 27, 2008
Where's the Lamb?

This would be referring to March, which is threatening to go out just as Lionly as it arrived.

I saw the Laser Lady yesterday, and she checked me off in the box that read, "No change from baseline." She keeps track along several categories of changes. This is a good thing, and I take no day for granted. I ended up walking a total of about seven or eight miles yesterday, which was lovely. And I slept really well. I'm ready for more!! So my energy has not taken a hit as of now.

Today I saw Acupuncture Man, and I had thought that I would need to be coming on a weekly basis now, but he proclaimed that I'm healthy and could wait 2½ to 3 weeks, which is when I'll finish with this round of treatment. I can always call if the heat seems to be building up in my system, or if there are changes.

I continue with my daily trip and have informed some of the staff about the BEAM ON salutation.

I have found that it is more difficult to slip under the radar with my new do. This is a double-edged sword, as I found out the other night.

We went to a Parker fundraiser—the Taste of Nashoba, where there were many restaurants, wine-sellers, etc. I snagged a thimbleful from my favorite brand of beer—Wachusett Ale—the company who created The Green Monsta, a new thing. Then I had to go back to try the Summer Ale, and the guy busted me.

"Uh—you were here earlier." What the hell? There were hundreds of people going through there, and he's keeping track of me? What's up with this guy's memory? And the cookie woman was no better. Okay, so I wolfed down a quarter of a chocolate cookie. When I returned for my one-fourth oatmeal cranberry sample, she scolded me.

So either these people have freakish memories, or my coif stands out. Or, they say that to everyone and I'm just taking it personally. They were joking, I'm sure. I guess I have moved from the Skinhead look, passing the baby chick look into something that needs product. Or color.

Even Nancy from Nancy's cafe remembered when I told her that I would be there for breakfast the next day with a friend.

She came out and greeted me, "You came here!"

I am just not accustomed to this. And the other side is greeting people who should know me, and having them just wave and walk on by. One woman recognized my voice and then turned around to greet me. This is entirely too much focus, don't you think? Me and my March hair.

And while we're discussing my vanity and self centeredosity, I have so far decided against earrings (or at least I haven't been able to bring myself to do anything) and I have taken up makeup. There you are. Among the Things I Have Control Over, and the Things I Don't, I am choosing to decorate in this way. It's nice that these are my biggest decisions in the past couple of weeks, and that I'm not figuring out my next surgical plan yet. Let's hear it for frivolous.

March 28, 2008
When Fair Isn't Fair

Referring to skin type here. My Laser Lady confirmed my theory that fair-skinned people tend to have more of a challenge with radiation. We're talking about skin that would be more susceptible to exposure, so that makes sense. Anyway, I luck out in this department, being swarthy as I am.

By the way, about the confusion around the gel/corn starch deal: No, I am not making a paste (pasties?!!). I've figured out how to apply the gel in a thin coat so that I do not need to use a hair dryer (or fan) to dry off. The corn starch is used later to eliminate any friction between skin and clothing. Think about how you would treat sunburn. You want to lightly moisturize the skin, and you want to avoid as much contact as possible between the skin and anything else. More than you ever wanted to know.

That would be the conclusion of fun facts for the day. The bank continues to be a source of hair fashion consult, of the unsolicited, albeit enthusiastic variety. Go figure.

Good weekend to all!

March 30, 2008
Out of left field

I went to pick up Kate last night. She had spent the day with a friend at the friend's sister's Destination Imagination tournament and then gone back to their house for the evening. We had dropped Kate off at school that morning, and being the trusting (or incredibly negligent) parents that we are, we waved as she got into her friend's father's car and drove off. I knew that he was wearing a red baseball hat (Kate is now telling me that in fact, it was an orange hat, from their trip to Tennessee last year).

The directions to the house were simple; they live a couple of towns away, but as I pulled into the new development, it was obvious which house was theirs. It was the only game in town, all lit up with half a dozen cars outside. I realized that other kids must be there, too, and that we had all arrived at the same time to pick up our children.

The storm door was closed, but the main door was open, and I could see Kate's frog sneakers among the pile just inside the door. I knocked. No response. I knocked louder and waited. Next I tried the bell. Still no response. A woman came and took something out of a small room just off the mud room. I waved, but she appeared not to see me. I tried the door, which I guessed might be open since they were obviously expecting people. It was.

I walked into the kitchen/dining room area, which was brightly lit, and around the table were a dozen or more adults. There was not a person under 40 in sight. They were clearly having a good time; there were lots of partially demolished dishes of food on the counter, and a couple of cakes on the table. No one said anything. I looked at them. They looked at me. I had no idea who the hosts were.

Time was suspended as they tried to register who this woman was who had marched into their house after 10 p.m., looking for all the world like she believed she had a right to be there, but who no one recognized. As I scanned the faces, there was one woman who looked familiar, but I could not place her. Their faces were an alternating kaleidoscope of confusion, utter surprise, wondering whether they should be worried, anxious, afraid, or angry. This is an incredibly entertaining mix of emotions, and seeing them in such variety on so many faces was an absolute stitch.

I felt like the Cat in the Hat in that place
Where so many strangers inhabited that space.

They looked at me with their inquiring eyes
Registering nothing quite more than a great big surprise.

"I'm Kate Stafford's mom!" I announced with a grin
And those faces relaxed, this was clearly no sin.

And who at that moment should suddenly appear?
But Kate S. herself, with Caitlin, her peer.

"She's gone again!" someone said with a shout,
As she stepped in closer to see what was about.

It was Caitlin's mama and then came her dad,
Why this really was not going to be quite so bad.

"We're having a party," (of that there's no doubt)
"Our team came in second, and now we are out,

But we had a great time, and we're still having fun
And hadn't realized that your Kate would be done.

So pull up a chair, and please have some cake
We're ready to finish this silly mistake."

But we needed to go, it was time to get home,
And I need to wrap up this long rhyming tome.

We made for the door, and you'll think I'm a nut,
But that lady I knew shouted, "Hey, nice hair cut!"

And so ends my tale of adventure last night,
With a hair-raising comment that made it all right.

It makes me chuckle every time I think of those stunned faces. I'm sure mine looked the same; there were just more of them. We did chat for a while, and I felt right at home with this friendly group.

Okay, that was it. More anon.

April 2, 2008
3/4

After tomorrow, I am three-fourths through this phase of the triathlon. I saw Laser Lady today, who pointed out that I am a little bit red underneath the arm. She said this is typical, as there is the most friction there. She brought me over to the mirror to take a look. I had not been doing my gel/cornstarch routine there, but will now. I do not tend to look at myself in the mirror with my arms up in the air, surprising as that may seem. I know that I talk to myself, but when I ask questions, I have dispensed with the formality of raising my hand to answer, and hence, I am not familiar with the underarm world. No self-pit-y here. It was Schoenthaler who pointed out that I have only eight more treatments to go, so I should be in good shape.

Gale mentioned that one of the administrators at the school asked her who had come to her parent/teacher conference.
Gale said, "Oh you mean my mom?"
The woman insisted that she knew what I looked like, and that it wasn't me. She thought perhaps it was an aunt of Gale's who looked like me. Hey, it's amazing how much like myself I look, Gale thought. I think she refrained from pointing this out.

My appointment with Hugs was cancelled because he went home with the flu yesterday. I'll see him Friday afternoon so that he can convince me to take Tamoxifen, and give me a prescription. My resistance is irrational; I just don't want anything else (I'm not going!), but I'm convincing myself to give it a try for six months, at least until my next surgery, and then reevaluate. It may be the long-termness of it that bothers me. By making it a less-than-forever commitment, it seems less intimidating. I can't put this thing totally away if I'm taking a pill every day, even though it is the pill that will help ensure that it stays away. Ah, there is no accounting for feelings sometimes.

April 5, 2008
Hugless in Emerson

The man was there. He was still recovering from the virus that had sent him home with a 103-degree fever on Tuesday (and made him feel more empathy with his patients who go through cycle after cycle of feeling lousy and coming back for more treatment to make them feel that way). He was back at work on Friday, clearly not quite in tip-top shape.

I registered at the desk when I arrived, and within minutes one of my favorite nurses from oncology came out, and said, "Okay honey, we're all set." I picked up my things and got ready to have my vitals taken, and she said, "Oh, not you, honey. I'm looking for him," and she pointed to a gentleman further into the waiting room.

"Oh, so now you're calling him, Honey, too?" I demanded.

She looked at me and laughed, and said, "Oh, Meg! You look great! So different! You need some gel for your hair, like mine." She pointed to her own purplish spikes. "I'll even get you some," she said.

I felt like a kid there (not to say juvenile, Duke reminded me…). That particular day there were mostly much older people, and the atmosphere in the waiting room was very quiet and somber as I bounced in, antsy to get on with my afternoon and get ready to celebrate Gale's 18th birthday.

The nurse came back a few minutes later, exclaiming how well I looked. I realized that she sees people at their absolute worst: nauseous, tired, discouraged, pale, and that it must be nice to see people when they return looking better. After determining that my weight, temp, blood oxygen, and blood pressure were okay, she showed me into a room.

When Hugs arrived, he did not, in fact, hug, but commented that I looked normalish. Normalish? That's a term I might use. He said that from where he sat, my hair looked kind of blonde. BLONDE? Is he BLIND? I know he was trying to make me feel better about its salt and pepperosity, but there was no need. That was just plain ridiculous.

"So, have I mentioned hormone therapy to you?" he asked.

"No, you have not brought it up even once," I replied. "I'm ready to roll with it," I added. (There should be some truth floating around in there, right?)

We discussed the possibilities of switching to one of the other medications after a year or two (Amitrex, Letrisole, or one other that I'm also not remembering fully), but whatever, we'll see how it goes with Tamoxifen first. The other medications are more effective when a woman is clearly postmenopausal, and because I was bumped into this state by chemotherapy, I'm in this in-between place, but not through the whole thing yet.

We decided I'd be back on Wednesday to have some blood work done when not in such a hurry, and that was it. He also checked on how the radiation was going and declared that I must have some Mediterranean blood to have so little effect on my skin. No hug on the way out, either, so I offered my elbow, and we bumped elbows as an exit greeting. I'll see him again in June to check on how the Tamoxifen is going.

I get bothered by all these freaking doctors' appointments. There are so many of them. I wish I could go through like at a car wash and have different things checked as I move along a conveyor belt. That would keep chats quick and cut down on return visits. Very efficient, don't you think?

About my hair: part of me wants to grow it down to my waist, and then decide if I want to cut it. I will never do that, and I may decide to keep it short, but it will be my decision, not a default happenstance, no matter how fortuitous in some ways.

Okay, I'm done ranting, and must get ready to go out for the evening. It was such a luxury to sleep in until 7 a.m. and not even get out of bed for another hour. I am not feeling tired, but I do think I'm sleeping more soundly at night. If that's the worst of the fatigue, that's a good thing. The radiation department is closed on Monday for installation of a new computer system, but there'll be six more treatments after that.

The sun came out!!!!

April 11, 2008
Countdown

I am glad that I am down to the last three rad treatments, including today's. I am starting to really be aware of the increased tightness, particularly under my arm. There is also some pinkness beginning under the boulder there. I can see where sweat and the rubbing of clothing would get very uncomfortable. I met with Laser Lady on Wednesday, which was my "discharge meeting" since this coming Wednesday should be my first day without treatment. She said to expect the effects of the radiation to continue right through next weekend, but that if I'm using moisturizer twice daily it should go away fairly rapidly after that.

She also said that many women experience a kind of letdown after radiation, particularly if it is the last part of treatment, because it has been a daily thing for several weeks, and there is such regular attention. Mostly it doesn't last more than four or five days before we figure out what to do with that time slot that was dedicated to radiation. I preempted this mini letdown by going ahead and having my rant earlier this week.

My target was the Great College Sort and its sequelae. This is proving to be a fascinating time of reexamining our values, how they are similar or different from Gale's, and how much we are willing to put our money where our mouth is. Duke and I have discovered that we are not, in fact, Gale, and that our own experiences of high school do not inform us about hers, or what is best/most desired for her. I graduated high school in a class of over 700, and attended a large state university. While I enjoyed both these experiences, I did not share the same kind of personal, deep commitment that characterized Gale's relationship to her student-driven charter school. My college, State University of New York at Binghamton, was highly ranked, and I knew that I would get a good education there. I had never really considered any other option. It was just out of the question financially.

We have even come to realize that our own view of her does not completely overlap with her own, and she has done her level best to make this clear to our rather thick-headed selves. We were certain that Gale would do fine anywhere, so we were in favor of a bargain financially. Gale was in search of the place where she could flourish, not merely "do fine." We have approached this situation with honesty, not to say stubbornness (well, maybe a little), and an intensity of feeling that matches the size of the decision.

I called Bennington College and said, "Hey, look pals. This is an oddball year for us, and my earning power is impacted by it."

They turned around and said, "Well, okay. We think Gale is the Bees' Knees, and what will it take to tip her decision our way?"

I said, "Jeez, we have always considered Gale to be the Bees' Elbows, and thank you for throwing yet another factor into this mix, and why don't you just transfer your endowment into our bank account?"

And that has stunned them into silence.

It may have something to do with the fact that Bennington is on their spring break right now, or are considering everyone else's requests, but we are waiting none too patiently to hear from them (maybe they haven't realized that the Bees' Elbows are much nicer than their Knees). In the meantime, Duke and Gale have gone today to revisit Purchase, which stands next in line in her favor.

We will see what all this brings. Time now to head out to my waning part-time job of going to Emerson. I will drop off my prescription for Tamoxifen on my way home.

April 14, 2008
Tears

After my last radiation tomorrow, I will be heading to Newburgh, New York, for the funeral/memorial service of our dear friend, Shirley Resnick. She and her husband were in a terrible car accident a week and a half ago, in which the vehicles burst into flames and left Shirley with a number of injuries. She had stabilized in the ICU, but developed sepsis and died yesterday. She and my mom started and ran a pre-school and kindergarten for over 25 years, and I grew up with her son, who is a month younger than I.

We watched stars together, made home movies riding their St. Bernard, and Shirley made my elegant pre-wedding luncheon (not a shower, she insisted). I said my first word in her presence (and have not stopped talking since). She had a unique clarity always about what she would or would not do, and you never had to worry about putting her out, because you knew she would give you the straight-up answer. I will miss her gentle, accepting presence greatly.

On a completely different note, but squashed into the same period of time, it's looking like we're closing in on a college decision. Bennington came through with some extra scholarship money. We're waiting on the official letter, and Gale and I will spend a day there next Monday taking classes. I'll bring my bike if it's nice out. If all that goes well, we probably have a deal. Last week was intense; our family discussion last Monday night resulted in extremely heated feelings as we weighed expenses against experiences, and preferences against possibilities and sacrifices. Gale went outside to her car in an effort to get some space. We would not allow her to drive in her agitated state and so she walked to her friend Anne's house in Pepperell. Twelve miles away. At night. We did not notice her cell phone in the driveway, but found it upon our return home at nearly midnight. To say we have all learned a lot is rather an understatement, but we have moved on, and are excited about Wednesday evening.

Still don't know if all this will distract me from the end-of-treatment letdown. Time will tell....

BEAM ON to all, and to all, BEAM ON!!

April 17, 2008
SPRUNG!! !

Life has been so dense the past few days it's hard to know where to begin. Yes, I am DONE with radiation, and active treatment!!!!! Okay, I'm coming back to repeat that news for anyone (like me) who might have missed it the first time around. DONE!! Tuesday was the last treatment, and I went racing out of there so that I could get home to meet my mom and her friend Gene to drive to Newburgh. The treatment went per usual, and then the nurse told me to halt the gel and cornstarch in favor of regular moisturizer of my choice a couple of times/day. A sheet of instructions indicated that I should not expose the irradiated area to sun for the next year, so…no topless beaches this year. I had seen some people receive little diplomas, which I did not, but it may have something to do with the speed with which I left the building.

At the service for Shirley, I was shocked to realize that it had been 10 years since I had seen my childhood friend Seth, Shirley's son. Herb (her husband) looked shattered, being exhausted both physically and emotionally. Their three sons were there with their collective children. It was wonderful to see all of them, and to see the way they treated each other and their dad. They were in almost constant contact with him and each other during the service, supporting one another as they each took a turn to speak.

The service itself was lovely. Shirley's niece, a close friend, my mom, and I each spoke before the three sons, and together we were able to convey a picture of this astoundingly spiritual, peaceful person who lived what she believed every day and cherished each moment of it. She had clarity about her life that was inspiring to be around.

Some of us have the good fortune of having people in our lives who are not parents, but who act as guiding influences and who help positively shape our lives. I was fortunate to have her there from the beginning, letting me know she loved me in ways both direct and indirect, and like many in her family, we benefited from knowing her. I feel sure that she was prepared and ready to accept her death with the same clear eye and ability to take care of herself that she brought to each day. I will miss her serenity and the way she championed my mom for more than 50 years. And I will miss hearing her swear, because although she conducted herself with grace and a certain properness, she could let out a good "what the fuck was that?" from time to time.

So that was on Tuesday.

I woke up on Wednesday and went NOWHERE!!! Instead, I could bake and prepare for Gale's dance performance. In between shopping and errands, I had a small window for a bike ride. It must really be spring!!

I needed to inflate my tires, of course, and I tried to use the "easy" foot pump, except that it required holding the tube in a way that was uncomfortable with my left arm, and I succeeded in deflating it quite rapidly. I tried a number of variations, absolutely determined that I was not going to be thwarted by the damn pump. I was getting quite a workout, and as I started screaming obscenities, Bobcat came strolling down to see who was joining him in one of his territories.

Completely unperturbed by my display, he climbed up on an old cushioned footstool, curled his tail around him, and settled back to enjoy the show. Did he offer up one paw of assistance? No, he did not. I should probably count that as a plus, because any assistance he might proffer would likely involve some kind of hairball. The hairballs that exit his body can hardly be imagined to have fit in there in the first place. I feel a further digression coming on, but I shall resist.

April 27, 2008
The Check Is In The Mail

At least soon, we hope. For Bennington, that is. It's been a continuing evolution and conversation, and it looks like it is leading this way. Got to be decided in the soon department, as the deadline for receipt of confirmation (backed up by some cash) is May 1.

I've made a new discovery about my toenails. Yes, that most comely body part that has been largely socked in the last several months. I had noticed a few weeks ago that my fingernails had an odd hue about them. I wondered whether I was making this up, but I have now discovered that my toenails have a definite line through the middle of them where the newer, healthier looking part is emerging. The top part has gone through some kind of Howard Hughes training, and looks disgusting. I pointed this out to Kate.

I could tell that she was prepared to reassure me that I was over reacting. She took one look, paused, and then said reluctantly, "Oh, you're right!" She clearly could think of nothing else to add, so she fled the bathroom. Not only is the top part a different color, it is a different (and less pleasant) consistency and texture. "Tell me more!" I can hear you saying. I know, who can resist a graphic description of toenails? Suffice to say that when I say Pedicure, I am emphasizing the cure part because otherwise I am stuck with these things that are really appealing only to Mr. Dog.

At any rate, I don't know if this is because of chemo or radiation, both, or some kind of peculiar bestowal from Middle Earth (or middle age). I'm just hoping that it continues to get better lest I scare my clients when I'm wearing sandals.

I'm pretty certain that my hair is trying to curl, but lacks the length to complete a full revolution. Instead, it's just sticking up in tufts; another attractive look. I keep talking about the product that I should put in my hair, and I better get on it or I'll look messy.

Yes! I have enough hair to look messy!

Duke has put in a plea for me to consult with my hairstylist (or the ladies at the bank) about how to have it grow in. I'll try to get it on my calendar.

I have been feeling really well. I've been out on the bike a few times and have put in up to 18 miles a couple of times, and around 14 or 15 others. Not speedy ones, but I'll get there for sure. I LOVE IT! I walked Mr. Dog today, because it is not fair that he should suffer just because I am biking.

The rest of life continues apace at the moment. Gale's second-degree black belt test was this morning, and she was awesome. The panel of fifth- to seventh-degree black belt-holders was very complimentary. It is sooo cool. I asked one of the moms how her older son is (he got his black belt with Gale a year and a half ago and is now in college).

She said, "Oh, he's doing really well...do I know you?"

When I told her that I'm Gale's mom, I worried for a second that she still didn't recognize me; but she pulled it together and made a nice comment about Gale, and then asked if Gale would be around this summer working at the dojo as she and her (the woman's) younger son had been last summer. Whew!

Gale's senior project presentation is on the 6th of May. Kate's gymnastics state competition is in a couple of weeks, and her soccer team is 3 – 0. Whee!

Duke and the girls made me an "end of treatment brunch/celebration" last Sunday: crepes, which we filled with different jams/ chocolate chips/ butter/ cottage cheese. Mmmmmm. Duke made one simple comment about being glad treatment ended, and I filled up and started to cry. I couldn't stop and I couldn't speak. Their three beautiful faces were looking lovingly at me, and then they started to look concerned, because they couldn't determine whether they were TOJ (tears of joy) TOS (tears of sadness) or TUO (tears of unknown origin). I finally managed to sputter out that they were a little of each. We had had a minor communication breakdown that morning, but nothing huge. I was glad and relieved to have the active part of treatment behind me. I'm hoping that I never have to go through it again.

I have worked so hard to have the treatment be not the main part of my life, not center stage, and yet here we were acknowledging the end of it. It has been a big deal, no matter how I slice it. And although I am thankful and grateful that I have come through intactish, it still has been a life-altering experience.

I am grateful to see my daughters continuing to live their lives, flourishing, and being themselves. And I am grateful that Duke has been willing to rub my arm and shoulder and listen to my various rants and complaints about having yet another appointment or about how my irradiated part has continued to tan or whatever. And I am so appreciative of everyone who has driven me, brought or sent food or flowers or books, responded to my e-mail, or just thought about the Breasty Business over the past nearly a year. Every single one has been received with my humblest thanks. It was right that there should be some nod to the end of this time. Sigh.

April 29, 2008
Done deal

Bennington is a lock. Yea!!

May 3, 2008
Twinkle Toes

And twinkle they do. I had a pedicure yesterday (my second ever, but clearly not my last!) and my toenails are now a gorgeous shade of red/orange. My feet have gone from drab to fab! They really do look better than ever, even by Duke's report.

My pedicurist also thought that some of the oddity was treatment related. It's the line across the middle that gives it away. A couple of people suggested that perhaps it was fungus (and where is the fun in fungus??). I may have been taking just the teeniest bit of poetic license when talking about them, but even Gale had to admit that they were pretty unsightly. Just trimming the nails helped a lot (less IS more here), but the pedicure really brought them to a whole new place (like Oz).

Plus, the chair you sit in while your feet are soaking in the bath, or being massaged, has rollers in it, so that by the end I'm pretty sure I was drooling and unable to put together a coherent sentence. The whole thing was thoroughly delightful, and now I think I should try out lots of different places so that I could do a report on which place is best.

The woman who did my last pedicure (I swear it was around 10 years ago) was also a dental hygienist. She liked doing both. I remember Duke making some comment about hoof and mouth; very disconcerting. She said that people white-knuckled their dental cleanings, but were relaxed for their pedicure. I guess you need to be fairly detail-oriented for both.

I did start taking the Tamoxifen, by the way. I couldn't be counseling my clients to take medication despite their misgivings when I know that mine can be helpful and not do the same myself. So far, nothing untoward has happened. It's only been a few days, but hopefully time will proceed uneventfully. I'm trying to think of it as daily protection, putting more and more distance between me and unwanted cells.

May 11, 2008
Curls just want to have fun

Moms, too! I neglected to comb my hair immediately upon coming out of the shower the other day, and it decided to do all kinds of wild things. I may have gone out of the house, except that I happened to pass by a mirror and yelped at what I saw. It really did resemble an ocean with the waves sticking up. I have to make a little effort to tame it into submission, and Duke thinks I should just keep it short (like my e-mails...um). I think once it grows down past my knees I will consider this. Or maybe not. I just haven't decided yet.

I had almost forgotten about my new hair status except that I wound my way through the building at work (because work is being done on the sidewalk, and we have this new labyrinthine route into the building) and arrived in the lobby to find an older gentleman hanging out there with a manila envelope (couldn't find any better company, I guess...). I asked if I could help him, and he said that he was waiting to see the lawyer, whose office is just off the lobby.

And then he said, "Nice haircut. Kind of different. I like it." And here I had been thinking that I had removed the sign that said, "Please tell me about my hair." But no! I'm beginning to get hooked on it. I'm going to have to seek out comments soon.

If all I'm chatting about is my hair, that must be a good thing. I do have an appointment with Plastic Guy this week. I'll be interested to hear what he has to say, if we're still looking at autumn for the next leg of my reconstructive journey. (No, I'm not switching body parts…)

My energy has been great. Earlier this week, Mr. Dog and I did our 3-mile constitutional, and then Ana and I did our first 20-mile bike tour of the season later in the day. It was awesome. Today I did a smaller version, because time permitted only 15 miles on the bike, but hey. You do what you can do.

Mom's Day was fun. Homemade waffles. The best. And it followed our meal last night in the North End, Boston's delightful Italian section. So much fun. More plantings in the garden (courtesy of Kate and Duke), and I am bejeweled with a homemade necklace from Gale and a fun bracelet from a very offbeat store in the North End. Lisa and Mom joined us for salmon this evening, and then we watched August Rush, which was a little predictable, but still fun, and with lots of music.

May 15, 2008
Corollary

I had a client this week who represents another take on the response to me and my (old) diagnosis. I had been thinking a few months ago that we did not really need to be meeting anymore, and was suggesting less frequent meetings, or talking about stopping. We did meet less frequently, but my client was clear about wanting to continue to meet. This is a delicate balance, and something that is open for discussion, but I do not want to insist that someone stop meeting just because I think he or she is ready. The client, too, needs to be ready, and it is not unusual for me to see someone's capability a little sooner than they believe it themselves.

I have had a sense about a few clients that they are being protective of me, and although no one has articulated it, I felt that part of their wanting to keep coming was out of a sense of wanting to keep track of me somehow, or make sure that I'm doing okay. Or something like that. Finally, this particular client had missed a couple of visits, and when we talked about it, at last acknowledged that part of the reason for continuing to come was wanting to make sure that I had a consistent client base, and that it was part of a way to contribute to my being okay. Our discussion about it freed him up to end treatment.

Today, another client was talking about a colleague who is undergoing breast cancer treatment and experiencing numerous side effects, some of them quite unusual and disruptive (including difficulty with vision). She has had to advocate for herself, switch treatments, etc. Another colleague is seven months into recovery and taking it easy. It was a reminder that I should not be taking those 20-mile bike rides for granted, or even my walking loops.

It does give me pause (and it gives the animals paws) to consider how much of my experience is absolute bull-headed insistence that I do not give up certain things in my routine and that I live my life as usual as much as possible. I don't want to think about it too much, and I will never really know what the balance is between good fortune, good care, attitude, and sheer ignorance about the (negative) possibilities.

What I do know is that whatever I experienced, it is my own, and that everyone has their own shade of gray about each aspect of treatment and their picture of it as a whole. I'm still too close in to really have the broad perspective yet. A colleague mentioned that she was looking for a therapist to work with a couple, one member of whom has breast cancer. Schedule apart, I declined to work with them at this time. A little space would be a good thing.

May 16, 2008
Here I Is....

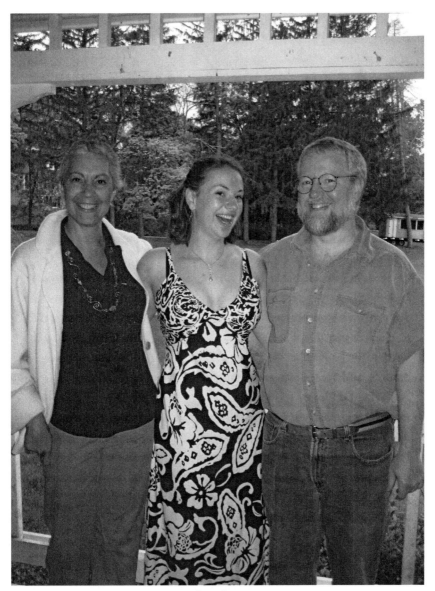

Prom Day

This was taken today at the gazebo in Littleton prior to Gale's prom. Will forward one of her and Nick shortly. Those kids could not look more terrific. A few of them prepped here at the house; God they're cute! So if I want to keep my hair really short, I will actually need a trim soon! Not sure about the gray. Maybe I'll try short and brown. I think I lack the patience to wait until it gets down past my knees before the trim.

So Plastic Office will be scheduling my Phase II surgery for either September 5 or September 19. Someone from his office will let me know. That will just be the swapping of the hard plastic tissue expander for the softer implant. Then, three months after that, there will likely be another surgery to slightly reduce Parton so that there is some reasonable match between them. My body is a work of art in progress (not to say a Wonderland, thank you, John Mayer). I knew there would be some more work, but now we're looking at December, optimistically, to have this thing done. This is not good for the impatient part of me, but again, there is nothing I can do but live my life and wait it out. The last surgery will also be the creation of the nipple from part of the reduction. It's all too weird for words, except oh ho! I seem to be using a great number of them.

May 26, 2008
Anniversary

It was last Memorial Day that I discovered the lump after my bike ride to Woods Hole from Falmouth. I knew that this was coming up, of course, and that we would again be on the Cape, and that it was likely I would be going for another bike ride. Which I did.

There's a lot that's different about being there. It is likely the second-to-last time, as Doug has signed a Purchase and Sale on the big house and the closing is set for June 28. We have been there without Val, and her presence is there, filling the space. The house looks much like it has, except if you open many of the drawers and cupboards, you find them vacant. Bob cooked us an awesome meal last night of Arctic Char and grilled veggies (can you say Heaven?). The kids made cookies, I walked the dog, many of the usual activities.

It was a beautiful day on the Cape, a full 15 degrees cooler than it is in Littleton. Duke and I set out for the 20-mile loop that takes you along the bike path near the ocean. People were out, but in nowhere near the numbers there will be in a few weeks. We were working hard, biking into the wind, pumping along, and loving it.

On the way back, it warmed up a little. The wind was moving us along and my mind was drifting. I can't wait to bike more on the Cape, or the Vineyard, or maybe we'll finally make it out to Nantucket. I'm thinking about the places I want to go with Gale this summer before she heads to Vermont. I'm looking forward to Family Camp with Duke and Kate and her friends Kate and Mal. It's all good, and it will be hard to make decisions about where to go when, the best kind of hard decisions.

It struck me that last year at this time I had no idea how difficult the decisions would be in the upcoming weeks. Memorial Day was the beginning of the unraveling of the blip that wouldn't end. It started small, with little concern on the part of my internist, but with the scheduling of my annual mammogram, and an ultrasound to follow; which led to the biopsy, and all the rest. The lumpectomy and pathology report would dictate the raft of treatment that would frame my year.

And now I'm looking back on it. I have the whole summer to consider swimming, biking, hiking, working, visiting, frolicking in a way that was not possible last year. We had a lot of good times last year, but it required more focus, more effort, and more help than I could have imagined.

My treatment has been like crossing a ravine on a narrow log. You have to look straight across and walk steadily without pausing or looking down, or it'll be scary, and you could lose your balance. The log is wide enough to cross, but you have to concentrate and resist the urge to glance down. By doing this, you are afforded a stunning view of the greenery around you, the sounds of the waters rushing below, and the scents of the wildflowers that surround the ravine. I'm on the other side, but I haven't really turned around to study what I have crossed.

There's more to come, after all, even if it is not treatment, but reconstruction oriented. Surgery is surgery, with incisions and anesthesia and more downtime. I need to get further onto the other side before I can turn around and take in the scene I have left. This anniversary date provided a sort of inevitable mirror, and I caught a glimpse of what we have come through without intentionally trying to look there.

Realizing that I have recently experienced the loss of three people from very different places in my life, has made me think about an essay that I wrote about three people whose deaths I learned about within a few months of each other, but who were not so close to me. Here is the essay followed by more thoughts as I continue to tread in this tenuous place.

Death is not convenient, sympathetic, or logical. It defies the expected, upends planning, and robs us of our confidence that we can anticipate what to expect; to say nothing of the pool of grief that can spill out and threaten to wash away our equilibrium.

In the past three months, I have learned of three sudden deaths: one in a car accident, one by a medical event, and one by suicide. I did not know any of the three people personally, but I know well at least one person connected with each loss. The abruptness in each case adds to the feeling of being off balance, not knowing exactly where it is safe to walk or what to trust. The notion of what is "fair" is so far out of range, it cannot even surface on the radar screen.

With the first two, neither person had done anything to stack the deck against themselves. No alcohol or reckless driving, no high risk behaviors. There is nowhere to point a finger and say, "Aha, I understand this." It is this measure of understanding that we humans so often seek to gain. In a landscape that offers no toehold of control, we try to ferret out meaning in order to absorb what does not make sense, what is so painful to integrate.

In all three instances, everyone has been cut off from the opportunity to say goodbye, to lay a chapter to rest in a way that makes for satisfying closure, even as the sadness wells up. There is nothing anyone could have done, and so the challenge is to accept the senseless, and try to integrate the shock into the fabric of life.

Each person must deal with the trauma in his or her own way. Community can gather and offer stories of celebration and consolation. In the willingness to communicate lies the possibility for connection, for healing in the arms of others.

This can soften the troughs of the roller coaster ride as the grieving wreaks havoc with schedules, sleep, concentration, and any sense of normalcy. Normal has been redefined, continuing to escape consistency or the familiar. Even when the old routine resurfaces, there is a missing piece, a sense of something elusive being askew.

There is no replacement for time in the continuum of healing, even as each person imposes a framework of religious, spiritual, and metaphysical beliefs in an important effort to structure the trauma. Poetry, music, and food can all be a balm, but it is not predictable when or what will be the most helpful at any given time. Solitude, too, plays its role in allowing us time to process without interacting. We must pay close attention to our mercurial needs during this time after the death of a loved one.

We are in some ways our most human in this vulnerable, raw state. As our increased sensitivity renders us open and subject to what is around us, we transform the pain of death and turn it into a connection with life. These stark contrasts, while unsettling, are all a part of the weave in which we live our daily lives. My hope for each of the three people reeling from sudden loss is that they are able to find crevices of light and hope surrounding the inevitable tender spots.

As I continue to absorb the loss of those close to me, and contemplate the fact of my own mortality, I remain unable to wrap myself around this reality; it simply does not feel close at hand. It is not that it feels impossible or too frightening in and of itself. I hope that I am able to address it when my time is nigh. I would not want to miss the opportunity to do this consciously. I just cannot go there when there is so much else that feels so pressing. Even as death is a part of the whole of life, I don't want it to take up space ahead of its time. If I can continue to focus on what is happening now, I afford myself the time to let in each event as it comes, put it in the best perspective I can. I cannot force more than this.

I want to be present for others when they face this, but do not feel it necessary to go there prematurely myself. As death is a part of life, so, too, is illness and other challenges. Breast cancer was one of mine. It wasn't the first, nor will it be the last. Each wave in its time.

May 27, 2008
Another First

I got my haircut today. Yep, an official, in the salon, full-on haircut. It was with Stephanie, who I really love. She is so normal. She's confident, clear, direct, upbeat, and very uncomplicated. She's 29, has two kids, and they are lucky because she knows what's okay, what's not, and she's not apologetic about letting them know. And oh yeah, she has used a pair of scissors once or twice, too!

She told me that as is typical, the sides have grown more quickly than the top, and that the first hair in is very downy. She barely trimmed the top, but took a little more off the sides, and gave me an actual haircut. The thing has an actual shape, and I like it!! We'll just have to see how it goes as it grows in, but I finally feel like it does not look haphazard, and is maybe the teensiest bit stylish. It feels neat (literally). Whew! And of course, I got just a tiny bit teary for a minute, just like I did yesterday on the bike ride.

Duke was asking me questions and I couldn't respond, and he finally asked me what I was thinking about; I had to pull over for a minute. My nose was already running, as is its way, and with my eyes running, too, I needed to stop for a minute and dry things up. There is nothing so lovely as hugging someone when you both have bike helmets on, tenderly crashing someone's chest with the dang things. Or just butting heads.

On Mother's Day, the girls were peering at me as I read my cards.

"I am NOT crying. Yet," I declared. I smacked my hand on the table and added, "I am not emotional!"

It is remarkable how ready my tears are to enter stage left and right at a moment's notice. Pisses me off sometimes. Who do they think they are anyway? What right do they have to invade without announcement? None, damnit. And they're so versatile, too. Ready to party for happy occasions, sad, new ones, unexpected ones. I'm a friggin' faucet. Must be I'm just limber. Facile. Agile with my emotions and in the moment. Yeah, that's it.

Anyway, I can finally say that my new look is created with some intent, not just by default.

June 2, 2008
Heart Throb

I came home this afternoon to a message from Hugs's office to call there and ask for Kim. It made me a little nervous because I was not waiting for anything. I have learned that news can materialize out of thin air. I called immediately to short circuit any undo anxiety and was rewarded with Kim herself answering the phone. I introduced myself to her, and she told me that she wanted to schedule me for an echo. This felt completely out of the blue (the only color for an echo).

"AN ECHO? AN ECHO? AN ECHO?" I wanted to ask. I suppressed two of them.

"Yes, Dr. Driscoll's office called to ask whether Dr. Dubois wanted you to have an echo before your reconstructive surgery in September."

I exercised yet more restraint and kept myself from shouting, "NO, I do NOT want an echo, echo, echo. I am perfectly fine. Better than I was before my last surgery, and that echo was perfect. I do not want another useless test, thank you very much."

This test is not painful, intrusive, or even terribly time consuming; I just do not want it interrupting my summer fun of bike riding, visiting, swimming, or even getting my next pedicure. Kim was being nothing but pleasant and helpful. And Driscoll and Hugs, clearly in cahoots, are being careful and conservative. These are good qualities in a physician, particularly when there is the time and no contraindication to do otherwise.

However, all I wanted to do was toss the phone across the room, out an open window, and into the bushes where it could take up residence with the remote control, which I have tossed out there a dozen times in my mind. Wow! Such a response from a seemingly innocuous request!

She was asking whether there were days that were better for my schedule than others. I should have suggested the week we'd be away, but instead brought it up as not so good a time. I conveyed my schedule to her, and she'll get back to me with a time.

My surgery isn't even officially scheduled yet. I need to call over there to push that process along. Just haven't gone there yet. I wonder why. Could it be that there's something I'd rather be doing? Like removing a splinter from my big toe? Or cutting Bobcat's nails? Or maybe cleaning up a hairball???? Could be.

I realized that I was holding an apple cinnamon rice cake in my other hand, which Kate had lamented was about as close as we get to dessert in our house at the moment (this was inaccurate; there are several dozen frozen Snickerdoodles snoozing in our freezer and a full bag of chocolate chips). Perhaps it was this lack of sugar that was affecting my mood, or my concern for my father-in-law. At any rate, even a rice cake offers some nutrition, and after eating it I felt a little more human, at least enough to rummage around for something else.

I'll have the echocardiogram, and there will likely be other tests that I will try to have scheduled for the same day for efficiency's sake. It will not be such a big deal. It's just that I have done a very good job once again of putting the next phases of treatment out of my mind, even if they are not "treatment," but reconstruction. It is still surgery, and we are not talking a finger splint. Being careful really is a good thing. I just hadn't been expecting that call yet. It came out of order: before I had the date scheduled, which is apparently the way I had been anticipating it.

I'm ready. It will not ruin my summer. I just needed a few minutes to get back on track.

Hope you're all loving this amazing June weather!

June 7, 2008
POOL'S OPEN

And the water is fine. Looks like it's actually going to be hot today, and the pool is begging to have its annual First Dunk!!!

The graduation was a particularly lovely and satisfying event. My mom had asked who the main speaker was going to be, and I replied that it would be 13 or 14 students, and 3 or 4 teachers. Any graduate who wished to, was given the opportunity to speak for two minutes (same amount of time speaking for the teachers, and the principal spoke for not much longer). This meant that there were all different essays about some aspect of the student's time at Parker or about graduating. It was personal, particularly interesting, and informative. Gale spoke, as did several of her friends, about leadership, relationships, leaving home, defining what personal best means (and for whom), being able to learn about and be themselves. The reception that followed was produced by the junior class, and we didn't realize how hungry we were until we caught sight of those appetizers and desserts. It was the perfect capping ceremony to their time at a school they all feel strongly about.

I had some thoughts about the whole process which I will forward at another time.

Looking forward to seeing those of you who can be here today and thinking of all of you who can't, particularly my father-in-law, who has been in the hospital with an intense fever and who continues to stump the staff of the ICU about what the hell is happening with his body chemistry.

June 9, 2008
Grad party etc.

Gale's graduation party was truly a lot of fun. It was HOT, but the tent provided by the Stockwells saved the day, especially when it rained. The enormous Whoopie Pie was a big hit (and the smaller ones were just as big in the hit department). Gale was particularly delighted with her gifts, which ranged from the sentimental to the practical, "Green" being a strong and welcome theme as well. It was a lovely capper for Gale's year. I do think that it'll take me some time to absorb that this is really happening, but I have all summer to get it.

Today I received a letter from Plastic Guy's office informing me that my son has been scheduled for surgery on September 5 at 3:30 p.m. Son? What son?!

Having opened the mail in the kitchen, my boys, Charlie and Bobcat, were of course in attendance. I looked at them and asked if they had been going for a different look that I was not aware of. I guess they would be called Moobs (the abbreviated version of Manboobs), but really, I was not so sure that this term applied to pets.

We did just spend a small fortune on Charlie because he contracted some bizarre thing that rendered him unable to keep anything down. Even though the vet gave him subcutaneous water to help rehydrate him, and it bulged off to the side, I was pretty sure that he was not looking for reconstruction to make this a permanent look. It did happen twice, but at different times, so it was not a balanced look anyway. And you know how concerned with looks dogs are. I'll call Driscoll in the morning and confirm that he still wants me to follow through with this thing and leave the animals at home. Perhaps he wants me to be more like them, and put hair on my chest.

Okay, I better get going if I'm going to get into the pool tonight. I can feel the motivation dropping like a pulled pork sandwich going down with a cold Corona.

Chapter 5

A Break in the Action

June 14, 2008
Going for Broke

Which in this case includes my hand. Nothing to do with poker. Just a few miles into our bike ride, I encountered a leaping curb. Don't you hate those? I did my Cirque du Soleil tryout right there, which Ana assures me was quite lovely. Just a little tumble with a roll, and I was back on my feet. Nothing to it, except that somewhere in there I must have whacked my hand because it was hurting a little.

I thought I took the brunt of the fall on my right shoulder, which is a little scraped up, and my right knee bears a little road rash. Somewhere in there I clearly knocked my hand on something, though. I made us go back to the car, where I fortunately had a little Tylenol/Motrin cocktail in my bag, and then we rode the rest of the 22 or 23 miles. My hand was starting to swell when we got back, and I went straight home to ice it.

This morning the swelling had migrated into the center of my hand, and the palm was starting to bruise, so I agreed to have it looked at. I went to my regular MD's office, who gave me an order for an x-ray, so when I got to the hospital there wasn't much of a wait. It was a good way to go, bypassing the ER. Sure enough, there's a break, and I won't know 'til I see an orthopod whether it'll be cast (in a supporting role), left with the brace that I have, or will need surgery. I'm hoping for whichever will leave me with the most mobility.

I swam a half hour of laps both yesterday and this morning, but they really don't want me using my hand. I'm going to have to take up jogging, or hope for a waterproof cast, or something. Jesus.

Clearly, my doctor visit quota was waning, and I needed to justify the reason I have decided to rent a trailer in Emerson Hospital's parking lot. The rest of me is a tad sore, too, and that massage gift certificate is looking pretty good.

This is not what I would call my lucky break. I think I will have to skip June next year. At least the middle of it. It doesn't seem to be working for me.

Enough typing. I'm trying to catch the multitude of typos since having to modify my typing style (I could get someone to do it with me, so we could be stereotyping). I still had a great time at the Punjab last night. Isn't it kind that they named a restaurant where I could justify my dubious jokes?!!!

Tomorrow we're Capeward-bound to see my father-in-law, who is home amidst the boxes before his move next week!

June 20, 2008
Breaking News

After consulting with the surgeon and taking a more informed look at the x-ray, I am electing to go ahead with surgery on Monday. The bone is out of line (so it better watch its step) and if left to heal as is, it wouldn't be terrible, but I would lose some strength in my grip. Some might say I'm already losing my grip, thus it's worth the surgical repair to regain whatever I can.

The best case scenario is for her to put in pins that would be removed in a month or so (they extrude from the hand—ick!). She feels this is not likely a possibility because the break is so high up in the hand, and there isn't enough bone to pin it to. Instead, she thinks I will probably end up with screws in there to realign it, and unless they bother me, the screws will remain (no jokes about my being screwed).

It rankles me to have to reschedule another day (at least) of clients, have my family rearranging themselves to cart me around, and face the possibility of another evening with Vicodin (to say nothing of the now predictable post-anesthesia roller coaster), but there it is. I do see this as a fluke break given the fall. My scrapes are pretty minimal, really. And given the length of time I've been riding, and the amount I ride, I have had very few injuries of any kind. It happens.

Still, this means another friggin' month with no swimming (even with a waterproof cast, there will be incisions, etc., and we don't want to invite any kind of infection), and probably no biking. We'll see. I will be walking my tootsies off, you can be sure. I just hope I'll be able to leave for Family Camp without any kind of apparatus.

On Wednesday, I saw both my Beam On doc and Hugs. Both feel I'm getting along famously (with what, I don't know). Hugs did happen to mention my dosage of Tamoxifen, and I realized that I'm taking half of what I should be (it's supposed to be twice daily and I've been doing once). Duke suggested that there might be something Freudian about this slip, but really, does Sigmund honestly have a place in my Breasty Business? I should think not. It just never occurred to me that the medication might be in any other form than once a day (you know how my imagination is so lacking).

Hugs was unconcerned about this little mishap, as I am only six weeks into a 5-year course of therapy. He was more worried that I would beat myself up about it, which I am not. I am not quite the perfectionist he believes me to be. I was able to set him straight, I think. If I can avoid self-flagellation about my biking antics, I surely won't worry about a little Tamoxifen. But I will take it correctly now. What's the point otherwise?

He had also wondered whether I felt like throwing my medication against the wall. Honestly, that is so immature. So much more fun to tap dance on those little pills and see which ones survive, don't you think?

Speaking of perfectionists, as we were, my typing is a tad fococta, and I'm trying to correct it, but I'm already slowed down by my splint and the inability to use all the fingers on my left hand, so I'm going to have to live with some of the typos.

By the way, a couple of weeks ago I had two calls in one day from clients with whom I have stopped meeting, but who wanted to know how I'm doing since they finished treatment before I finished mine. Isn't that sweet?

June 23, 2008
In the Loop

That's where I am and thought you should join me. Back to Percocet for the time being, although I may reopen my pharmaceutical wonderland for tomorrow.

The surgery was a little more complicated than anticipated. She tried to do the pins and that didn't work, so she tried to put in screws and that shattered the bone, so she ended up using wires and then pins and referring me to a hand specialist, who I will see on Wednesday. I, who embrace the direct and simple, am having to travel the complicated and circuitous. Hopefully, not too complicated. We'll see. We are talking some very small bones here.

There have been some questions about bone density. I will have this checked, but my hand was black and blue on my palm, and on two fingers up to the second knuckle. It was whacked hard. Ana even declared that since she witnessed the entire routine, she was actually relieved that I did not do more damage to my shoulder or collarbone, and was further relieved that it was only a little bone in my left hand that ended up hurt. I took a good tumble; this was not a little tap resulting in a break.

Starting to get sleepy. As usual, the nurse at the hospital gave parting instructions as I was swimming desperately to break the surface of consciousness. It's such a challenge to focus (uh-oh); that's why they write things down. I hopefully had not been dwelling too long in Freud's territory.

Just to have something non medical…we dropped Kate off at camp for three weeks at Rowe! Braces off on Thursday, last day of school on Friday, buds over to swim on Saturday, and then Campward she went!

Mark sent us a card with a duck on the front, and a message on the back about how the duck represents one of the signs of the I Ching, the book of changes. The Duck is an unfettered spirit, meeting fortune's unexpected turns with growing equanimity. I think I should follow one around for awhile.

Must be prone now.

June 25, 2008
Consult with the Hand Man

The following was sent to Steve, Susan, and George's friend who is a hand surgeon in the Richmond area.

I saw Brunelli (hand specialist) today, and liked him a lot. I felt he was clear, straightforward, and informative. He did take more films, but they're not on disc, thus they are not included with the ones from surgery and before, which I sent today. He seemed puzzled by a lot of things, starting with the timing of when I had the initial x-ray, consult with the orthopod, and surgery. He said that he would have been inclined to do *nothing* but stabilize after the initial break.

Dr. Kim did present that as an option, but it was clearly the lesser option. She was concerned that leaving it on its own, it would leave me with a weaker grip, and that the repair would help ensure a return to more normal functioning. So although I would always prefer the least invasive route, I opted for the best functioning, and therefore, surgery.

Brunelli also said that if he had done the surgery, he would have gone with a different type of splint, allowing for much faster mobility, so that by the time it was removed I would be almost back to normal, whereas this way it will be stiff and take more work to get there. He rewrapped it firmly and referred me back to Kim, who I will see on Tuesday. He also said that rather than using pins, he would have put in a plate if the screws failed.

My inclination is to see Kim for the follow-up, then switch over to Brunelli. I question her judgment in not referring me in the first place and then again in how she handled the surgery. I don't want to make myself crazy with what-ifs, and I want to move forward in the best way possible from here.

I'm hoping that the bottom line is that my hand will be fine; I'll be back biking and using it just like I have been. It is truly unfortunate that I have to wade through this medical mire now, but c'est comme ca, that's how it is. Thank you for taking the time to check this out; I really appreciate it. My medical education has been a little too encompassing this year.

June 29, 2008
South paw lore

So there has been a rumor circulating that my left hand has spent the last several years dwelling in the bottom of a Cheese Puffs bag. This unjust explanation for the luminous color of all the fingernails on my left hand was probably started by my right hand, which is a rather mundane pinkish tan color. Even the indigo hue emanating from the rest of the fingers does not seem to convince my more conservative right hand that the left one has not been having more fun.

I've overheard the left one threatening to unwrap itself and show the right one the pins protruding from its back. I have discouraged this display, given my extremely high squeam quotient, and the likelihood that I will faint immediately. My left hand, still irritated, is unmollified. It will likely next threaten to hurl me into a "Walk Like an Egyptian" routine, at which I am now quite adept. I am pleading for a truce between them and increased communication, as we know how fruitful this can be. The left's bandage is currently basic white and huge.

I am having to negotiate this single-handedly, as no one else will step in. If my right hand will promise not to cast aspersions on its fellow digits, I'm sure the healing will continue without handicap. Okay, I think I've nailed this one.

July 6, 2008
Cranky Panky

My x-ray last week showed that nothing had shifted, and I'm hoping for the same this week. It's pretty set after about three weeks, so pin removal is likely to happen next week, before the pins can turn into little conduits of infection, which I'd like to avoid. Instead, I march about like the statue of (non) liberty with my arm in the air. People have begun to offer encouragement during my walks to keep it upright.

"If you keep it in the air, it won't throb," one guy offered.

The woman on the bike just suggested I keep it upright without further explanation. Maybe I should combine this with hair consultation.

At any rate, I'm hoping I'll be able to head off to Family Camp with a less bulky splint than the number I'm sporting now. I won't be able to do the hikes that involve ladders unless there are people (whose name is Duke) who want to push or pull as I edge along. I'll just have to discover new trails.

When I saw the surgeon and laid out everything the specialist said, she was very apologetic. I told her that the bottom line is that I should be fine, just will have more work to do to regain full range of motion. She became teary. Tears actually came down her face. She said that she had done a number of these and that this had never happened before. I don't know if I had been expecting her to be defensive or dismissive or matter-of-fact or what, but I was not prepared for her to allow her vulnerability to show so much.

I was trying to let her know that I know she did the best she could, and she was telling me that "It's your hand; it's your life!" It was a weird scene.

My doctor friend Susan's point is that she should not have been doing it if she was not prepared to deal with this possibility. Gale said I should write her a note telling her she's a compassionate human being, and then switch my care. Very succinct, don't you think?

July 9, 2008
Castaway

Among Duke's lesser known talents is his latent nail clipping ability. It was actually me who performed the clippage when it came to the cats and most of my own nails. Duke had to step in and help out when it came to my right hand.

I now understand the cats' irrational reluctance when it comes to this non-painful act. It seems like it could be painful, so the tendency is to avoid it at all casts, I mean costs.

I am PISSED OFF that I am stuck with this thing for longer!

I was also reduced to tears on Sunday when I was vacuuming out my car, got really hot and just wanted to jump (or walk carefully) into the pool. But couldn't. It just got to me. I did go for a walk, which helped. Anyway, my Echo ECHO ECHO went fine this morning.

I'm finding that I can go back to typing with 1½ hands, which is so much better than just one, and I've been compiling a categorized list of things that are tricky with one hand (like dental flossing) or just a pain in the butt (like bringing in groceries). I think I'll go do some cooking.

July 12, 2008
BEAR ESSENTIALS

We picked Kate up from camp today, who told us about the bear that had been seen near camp on several occasions. Evidently, there was one morning when the blueberry buckle (Kate has told us of the widespread renown of the buckle) was being served, that the bear came close to the kitchen. The cook, who evidently packs mace in the kitchen, deployed it at the bear. This set off coughing fits throughout the dining hall.

And the bear, who obviously arrived hungry, left eMaciated!!!!! Haha!

July 16, 2008
Handyman Special

I am relieved to be solely under Brunelli's care now. I walked into his office and the staff was oogling my cast, asking where I got it, commenting on how pretty it is. Some people wondered whether I had done the artwork on it. Evidently, they had a hard time convincing the surgeons there to even get colors for casts. So old fashioned; they need to get with the hip program of fashion casts.

I found a seat in the second of two small waiting rooms, and realized that the very petite woman sitting next to me was wearing a huge tee shirt that read:

Things To Do Today:
Get Up
Survive
Go Back To Bed

Shit. I wanted to run away. I was in orthopedics. We got our injuries *doing things* like bungee jumping and skate board tricks, and complicated computer gyrations. This woman sat quietly, but her intensity rose off her like heat from a grill. I got out my book and stuck my nose in. I did not want to partake of her negativity.

Soon a man came in and sat down, and the two clearly had seen each other there before. They started chatting about their respective experiences, and each of them was dealing with a chronic issue— multiple surgeries, residual pain, unresolved issues.

I did not want to let this in. I absolutely could not consider anything that might result in anything ongoing. I want this open, shut, done.

The tight quarters of the room fostered conversation, which I did not feel like having. I was not ready to be dealing with a whole new set of personalities, but when the nurse came in, Ms. Tee Shirt came to life and was joking with her, animated. They politely asked about my injury, and I gave them a brief synopsis (yes, I can do that).

I was finally ushered into a patient room. It was a relief not to have to disrobe to be seen. Brunelli swept in, pointed out that the outrigger my cast was sporting is obsolete, and asked his assistant to free me from it and take x-rays. She got out her little saw and eventually removed it. The saw made me nervous at first, but it is a bit like clipping nails. It does not hurt, but looks like it could, so you have to fight the urge to tense up. He removed the tape around the pins, and I inadvertently caught a glimpse of them, but managed not to faint.

Then we looked at the x-rays. He doesn't think there's been enough growth in the bone to even consider removing the pins. I chose the color purple for my new cast, which will remain on for at least three weeks, at which time I will return for a visit. At that point, we will discuss what happens next. I'm really hoping to avoid his going back in to put in the plate that he would have put in had he done the surgery in the first place.

Bernadette had commented that Brunelli is a big guy, like a line-backer. I had not recalled this from my first visit, but I did notice this time. Do you think that the Percocet haze had anything to do with my perceptions?!

Please direct any healing thoughts to the bone in my hand. This cast is much more expertly done, a much sleeker line, bright purple, with the two fingers above the bone immobilized by the cast. Sigh. So off to Family Camp we go on Saturday.

July 27, 2008
Overcast

I was able to hike just fine with the cast, with the exception of the Beehive, a favorite hike involving ladders. I enjoyed the alternative hike that day, and know that there will be many Beehives in my future.

I only dunked in the lake once, but fortunately it was not a heavy swimming week because of the weather. Next year I'll be in there daily. It is not easy keeping your hand in the air as if proposing a perpetual toast.

My cast makes for a conversation piece, but after awhile I'm certain that people are just being exceedingly polite, because really aren't they stifling yawns? Gawd, surely she cannot be going on about that thing Again.

Duke began to worry when one day the conversation between my cast hand and right hand took another surly turn. It was the on the way down from the summit on the rainiest day, when I realized that my 20-year-old raincoat was not, in fact, doing its job. I donned the pair of long Subway sandwich bags (perfectly shaped for a cast) and stuck the whole deal into my raincoat sleeve. My left hand started up its diatribe.

Left hand: "Let me out of here!"

Right hand: "No way! You need to stay dry! I'm doing all the work around here. All you have to do is stay dry!"

Left Hand: "I do, too, help. How do you think those hiking boots got tied?"

Right Hand: "So what. Just stay in the bag and keep quiet!"

And so on.

Is it any wonder that I decided to jog down the entire trail? It had stopped raining enough to take the whole thing off when I got to the bottom. I started to treat them like puppets, and even I realized I was going around the bend.

Last night I started feeling like crap, and have been running an increasingly high fever over the course of the day. I'm convinced that I have an infection brewing somewhere. I thought it might be my hand, but I'm now actually wondering if it's related to my Breasty Business. I have many appointments this week, but Plastic Guy did call in an antibiotic. Hand Man was reluctant. He doesn't know me well enough to know that I would not ask for anything unless I really felt I needed it. We'll see. I have been completely lethargic today, coming around some with Tylenol or Advil. A fever higher than 100.5 is more than I've had since last year.

Duke just returned with Keflex. These bottles are clearly not designed for people with a cast on one hand. Here's the antibiotic to make you feel better, but first a little quiz on how creative you can be to break into the bottle, just to see how far we can push your sanity. "Bite me!" it seems to scream.

July 30, 2008
Balance

I know that this is not exactly news, but my experience this week brought home the importance of combining personal expertise with that of the care providers. My plastic surgeon performs and checks on surgery every day, many times a day, so he is in a much better position to know what to expect from the general population. I can't have a beat on what is typical, or within expected limits. He has a better read on what can be concerning, or should be attended to.

On the other hand, I know my own body and what is typical for me. I have a keener sense of when something is off, even if it may not be off for someone else. He commented on the slight redness around the surgical area, which he was not concerned about because it is not unusual for irradiated skin. However, I know that it was likely an indication of something going on for me because it is not how it has been these past several months. That redness is new and warm. He felt better knowing I would continue my Keflex, and I'm glad I am, too. I don't take anything if I don't need it, and he is aware of that. The collaboration between physician and patient is most powerful when there is the trust for each to hear the other. Each view is critical and cannot screen out the other.

Today's adventures in medical land brought the bone density test. I'll get results for this simple, non-invasive test next week, and am glad it is not the bonehead density test. Though useful, I can see the potential for abuse.

Hope you're enjoying this gorgeous summer day. I'm back on the walking trail, and Mr. Dog is wagging his fluffy tail.

August 1, 2008
Well Appointed

I saw Andrea Reciniti yesterday, my little firecracker of a surgeon. She asked about my hand, of course. As soon as I mentioned Brunelli, she lit up. He seems universally respected.

When she learned that he may need to go back in to put in a plate, she said, "Oh, if you need a plate, it'll be fine."

Perhaps this casual attitude is a good one. Yeah, just a little more surgery. What's a little incision and anesthesia between friends? What the hell? What would I be doing anyway? Working? Riding my bike? Shopping for college? Living my life? Details.

I don't want my surgeries colliding, though. September 5 isn't that far away for the next leg of my reconstructive journey (not really a leg, as I mentioned).

She also commented while checking for fluid retention in my limbs that I still have a bruise from my bike fall two months ago.

"Oh, no," I assured her. "That was from last week when I bumped it while tromping on gigantic boulders around an island in Maine." I hadn't really paid attention after the initial egg went down. It's a 6-inch bruise now.

She shook her head a little and said with a smile, "You're a piece of work." Hot damn! When was the last time your doctor called you a piece of work? Wasn't that sweet?

And since we're talking about unusual compliments, we were sitting at lunch one day at camp. There were several of us, as always. The tables seat nine. We must have been talking about age, because I said mine, and Tom A. looked genuinely surprised and said, "Really? Well, you don't ACT it!" How lovely is that?!

Got my blood work back today, and it's awesome. My cholesterol hasn't been this low for years. Now I'm just waiting on my bonehead density.

August 4, 2008
Hair of the dog

Think Schnauzer, which is what my hair most resembles now. Shapewise, I may have even crossed over into Poodledom, but the coloring is more Schnauzer. I haven't brought this up in the past 2½ minutes, but Duke and I were looking at photos that we have on the computer, and I became really aware of the changes in my hair. A couple of people have mentioned to me that they look different to themselves in photos than they do in the mirror, and now I understand what they mean.

The first hair back in was very fine and straight and mostly silverish. I guess as it continued to fill in, more pepper was added, and somewhere in the past couple of months the curl came back with a vengeance. Kate may have been the one at the Sox game yesterday, but my hair is doing a big-time wave. Jane noticed a difference between June and now.

I can't tell you how odd it is to have my hair making all these changes without the aid of chemical intervention, or asking permission, or anything. I guess technically it *did* have chemical assistance, just not the topical kind. I still don't know how I feel about coloring it or not, cutting it or not, but until I have a sense of where it's going to settle out, I'll just continue my wait and see. And I'll try to get used to the new look, which mostly I hadn't minded until the photo thing. Weird.

Tomorrow, the fate of my hand rests in the Hand of Fate. I figure best case scenario is cast off and splint on for a couple more weeks. Next best would be cast on for a couple more weeks, and least pleasant would be more surgery. This is where surprises are not so welcome, but who knows?

August 5, 2008
In the Pink

Which refers to my new cast color. The x-rays showed not enough bone growth to remove the pins, so he recast it, and I'll go back on the fifteenth for pin removal. It's possible that there is growth but that it's not showing up yet. The osteo evidently doesn't show well, but when it becomes calcified, it does, so we're giving it some more time. At that point, I'll get a splint and start therapy, and that will either promote more growth or it will fall apart. So we're protecting the investment I have made in this fix and hoping that the extra time will help make the difference. It certainly doesn't make sense to jump to more surgery at this point. I'm hoping not to go there at all.

I picked Kate up from gymnastics yesterday. It was her first time back since June, so when I walked in, her coaches exclaimed about my cast and asked what happened.

"I was bungee jumping in the Grand Canyon," I told them.

By the astounded looks on their faces I could tell that they bought it, but I am a pathetic liar, so I immediately backpedaled and came out with the truth—the briefest of versions lest Kate break into a wail right on the spot.

At any rate, I think pink will accessorize nicely with the dress I am wearing to my brother-in-law's wedding on Saturday. We can't wait. It should be a blast. Their excitement is contagious.

I was prepared for today's appointment, so although the result was not the best case scenario, it wasn't the worst, either. My family prepared a kickin' birthday meal and cake for my return, so it may have taken awhile to get there, but it was a delightful celebration nonetheless. Salmon, potatoes-and-onions on the grill, and salad. What else is there (besides homemade chocolate cake)? I will waddle to bed happy.

August 11, 2008
Cast of Character

Mark and Laurie's wedding was a delightful outdoor affair. There were kids playing ball, families picnicking, and our wedding party near the river. Mark's friend emceed the event, down to the pronunciation of wife and husband, by the power invested in the Justice of the Peace who hadn't arrived yet, and the community present. Then we shuttled off to another park with a restaurant for the dining and partying part of the evening. How fun to be immersed in the combined community of friends and family of these two adults who orchestrated the entire day with precision, flair, and a love for each other and all of us.

We arrived home to find my bonehead density results, which the paper indicated were "normal." I hadn't realized that I had been holding my breath a bit waiting for results. Is that why I'm blue in the face? It does take some energy to make sure that I'm not trotting down the path of false assumptions or negative outlook. Maintaining focus is a conscious act, and one that has become habit in many ways, but there are times when it takes more effort. I forget that from time to time.

One of my clients asked me today how I keep my outlook. I was startled at first, because I don't usually think about it so actively. I'm fortunate that I am genetically programmed in a glass-half-full kind of way. Actually, calling it half full is a load of crap; I keep my glass topped off whenever possible. It's less effort, and a hell of a lot more fun to focus on the good stuff. The hedonist in me demands it.

August 17, 2008
Cast-off

Well, the cast came off and the pins were removed. My arm no longer looks like a stringed instrument (does that mean I no longer need to fret?) and Duke is out of danger of being inadvertently bonked in his (and my) sleep by a pink cast.

I got a little squeamish around the (rotisserie-like) pin removal, and also when looking at the subsequent x-ray, which showed, at a minimum, nine holes in the metacarpal bone. Jesus! What was she doing in there?

The assistant was pointing them out and counting them, when she suddenly pulled up short and suggested that maybe it wasn't helpful to add them up. I think that was when I asked for a glass of water as a way to deal with the increasing squeam factor. It made me realize the level of trauma that went on during the surgery and clearly accounts for some of the swelling that is still evident in my paw.

At any rate, the x-ray also showed no movement, which makes Brunelli more hopeful that my hand will come around with therapy and will hopefully not need surgery. He also felt that I didn't need to have a splint made for it, because it would only be for protection and would slow down the limbering up of my fingers.

He asked me to straighten them as much as possible and then make as tight a fist as possible. They couldn't get up higher than a 45-degree angle, or much lower than that, either. We were talking about a follow-up appointment, which was looking to coincide with my next Breasty Business surgery.

I mentioned this, and Brunelli said, "So, wait. You're dealing with two major things here." Well yeah, I guess.

I can be as aggressive with therapy as I can tolerate, which at the moment means I am using my 45-degree fingers to type. Man, are they stiff. It is weird to have a part of my body be so unresponsive to the messages I am sending. I can see them glancing up at me, saying, "What, are you crazy? You want me to curl? Make me!"

Last night's activity was peeling off the dead skin while watching the Olympics. This totally grossed out Kate, but was immensely helpful in getting my hand to look semi-normal, aside from the swell state it's in. With the dead skin cover, they looked kind of like a fake lizard accessory. My pinky and ring finger are still veering left a little bit, trying to recapture that Live Long and Prosper posture that was so easy in my cast state. Have you ever tried to do a thumbs-up in a cast? Rock on works better, tubular better still.

So I was at the desk, checking out, making my follow-up appointment, which happens to be earlier on the same day as my Breasty Business surgery. Another office person called the occupational therapy office and was making those appointments when my cell phone rang. I shut off the unfamiliar number while considering the preponderance of frigging appointments.

"These are a lot to fit in," one office person sympathized.

"You have no idea," I assured her.

Checking my message outside the office, it turns out that my surgery has been moved to earlier in the day, so I marched back into the Handy office to change my follow-up with him. This overlapping of medical issues bumps up my insanity quota, especially since, starting the last week in August, we're back into carpooling the kids to school.

I'm hoping that once I get the routine down with Occupational Therapist, I'll be able to do most of it myself, and not have to spend more time at Emerson. I swear they should give me a frequent buyer card so that I get every sixth co-pay free.

August 23, 2008
Outcast

The first sobering experience was visiting with our friends, the Bronder-Giroux family, two days after my cast came off. We had seen them the night of my initial fall, when my hand was swollen and a little painful, before we knew it was actually broken. When we saw them last week, my hand was swollen and stiff (and we are not talking lucky stiff). It has been nearly 10 weeks in between. Have I traveled all this way only to end up in the same place?!!

I have to remind myself that although in a more difficult spot, it is in the service of renewal (hopefully). Two points in a tunnel can be equally dark, although one may be miles from the end, and the other is around the bend from the light.

When I saw Pat, my Occupational Therapist (which really sounds like a Career Counselor), she started my hand in the whirlpool bath. We then worked our way through a series of exercises designed to stretch my tendons and coax them back toward their natural shape and working ability. She is clear, direct, willing to push me, and willing to chat, a good combination for me. However, it was another slap upside the head to remind me that this is going to be a long road of therapy and work in between appointments.

I realized that I had been minimizing what I thought I would need, figuring that I could go to a couple of appointments and then work it at home. Wrong. She can use both hands to stretch mine, and impose more discipline than I might, no matter how much I'm using my hand and trying to do the half a dozen exercises half a dozen times a day. So I'm signed up for the next several weeks, as far out as the computer would allow.

I have already used the analogy in my therapy practice of needing to make the time for the treatment if I really want it to get better. It may happen on its own, but much more slowly. Intent and focus, the vital ingredients once again. I need to get my butt over to O.T. for help from the expert. I cannot take everything into my own hands.

It's getting better. I can type much more easily than last week, although it is still a long way from straightening out or making a fist. Maybe it's a good thing that my next surgery will overlap my hand therapy. I am pawing at the earth, ready to address different challenges professionally, but clearly I need to focus on my healing and get my body in order first. When I can focus on the big picture, I know that this will be just a short time, a mere plink in the bucket. It is when I become mired in some of the day-to-day challenges that I get frustrated. It is fortunate for me that I can shift back and forth; sometimes it is difficult to keep up. The Now takes on such a large presence that it fills the frame for the moment. That's when I need to get out and walk, or visit, or babble to you guys.

We are in prep mode for the launching of Ms. Gale for Bennington next week. She has taken advantage of these last weeks to visit with friends, buy enough stuff for the next century, and prepare for the great adventure. Ye ha!!! I am excited for her, even though I know I will cry my way back through Vermont after we leave her.

It is a spectacular summer day, beckoning me to come out and play. Who am I to refuse?

Chapter 6

Reconstruction

September 1, 2008
Launched

He stood poised, pad and pen in hand, ready to take my order.

"What'll it be?" he queried. "Percocet? Vicodin? What's your pleasure?" Wasn't this like ordering dessert before the meal?

"I think I still have some from last time," I replied.

He waved a dismissive hand. "Probably out of date."

We settled on Percocet and moved on to the rest of the appointment. I had already initialed 10 pages of information about the surgery on Friday, so I was pretty much up to speed on all the possibilities—large and small—of what might happen. For example, I knew that this might result in further surgery. Plastic Guy also wanted to make sure I remembered that after this, there would probably need to be one more procedure to balance things out.

He had said this from the start, so there was no expectation on my part that this would be the end.

"So, I'm agreeing with myself," he said. "That's good."

I have to say, I'm in favor of consensus among my surgeon. When there starts to be dissention and arguing in a cast of one, we need to worry.

A warning: the next paragraph may be Too Much Information for some of you. If that's so, you should be sticking your fingers in your ears and saying LALALALALALALALALALALA until it's over.

Anyway. The balancing will happen in a few months, most likely. This will involve Parton, as Dolly's irradiated skin can stretch only so far. When he swaps out the hard plastic expander for the softer, more drapey implant, Dolly will likely end up a little smaller than her counterpart. Therefore, the slight reduction will have to be given up by Parton. It is at this time that the nipple creation happens with tattooing and I think a little extra skin. At any rate, I am expecting that after a few days, not only will I be returning to work, but I should feel much more comfortable. Duke is anticipating that I will want to walk my loop by Saturday. We'll see.

This weekend, I'll be on the Percocet Cruise, which could be a boon for my finger exercises. I have discovered that as much as I love exercise, the ones for my fingers are really not so fun. It's mostly about stretching to the limit of pain, and honestly, I'm not so big on that. I'd fail miserably at Masochism School. But if I'm sailing along on Percocet, I could probably extend this particular barrier. So, if I actually remember to do the exercises, I should make great strides. By the time I see Handy Man on the 9th, I'll have made even more gains than I already have; it is improving; I'm just impatient.

And then there's the issue of hair, of course. On my hand. I was pointing it out to Duke yesterday.

"Wow! That's hideous!" Duke commented.

"Hey, Duke, thanks for weighing in, Pal."

"Wait, let me see," requested Kate. I showed her.

"OoOoh," she replied, aiming for tact with limited success.

"Nice, guys," I said.

Then they started backpedaling.

"It was the way the sun was hitting it just now."

"I hadn't realized that the hair was so dark."

Yeah, right. I took a razor to it in the shower, but really, it feels very weird. Duke brought out his teeny electric clippers and offered up a trim, but my arm was wet, and that didn't seem so smart.

We delivered Gale to Bennington on Thursday. It was a gorgeous day, and as soon as her roommate arrived it all fell into place and felt right. We unpacked, had lunch under the tent, and Duke and I went to hear a student panel speak while Gale and Kate hung out in her room. They were great speakers, each one with a different experience, but each was articulate and appreciative of their time at Bennington. We were going to wait to hear the president give a little talk as a Farewell to Families, but it felt like time to leave, and so that's what we did. We'll hear her next month at Family Weekend.

Gale was ready. She had done a great job preparing herself, seeing people, checking off her list of things to do and put behind her. All that remained was to make the leap.

By doing this, she had prepared us as well. She has been increasingly independent the past year, driving herself everywhere and making her own plans. We made a point of scheduling time with her, because we all need that contact. It is part of the nourishment that sustains our family. I have complete confidence in her making this transition. It is not that it will be without bumps and challenges; it is that I know she has the tools to handle them when they arise, and will ask when she hits bigger barriers.

It is characteristic of her that she fully embraces wherever she is, and I know that she will do this at Bennington as well. Finishing up business as much as possible is what has created this space. I miss her, of course, and know that we will develop a new rhythm of contact by Skype and text and phone when she is in a place with service. I am eager to hear about all the new adventures. It will take some time for this new status to sink in; so far, it has only been a few days, and I can fool myself that it is like camp. It is little moments that produce tears. When Nick left the night before we brought Gale to Bennington, my heart broke for them; but it is clear that they will stay in touch and remain close, working this anticipated separation as best as they can.

At any rate, I am enjoying my last days in the pool for this year, watching Kate do her own preparations for school, which has already begun, and enjoying the visits with friends as we watch the light begin to fade a little earlier every day.

Catch you on the other side of the double-edged scalpel.

September 5, 2008
Perky-set

Hey guys! I'm HOME!!! I got back 15 minutes ago, which exceeded even my hopes for a return time. By the surgeon's report via Duke, everything went well, and he thinks I'll be pleased. I will stay ahead of the pain today with my Percs of the day, and see how it all goes. What I would really love to do is swim, but that is not such a good plan for today.

Wheee! I am relieved to have this part done, and I will check back in with Plastic Guy in a week.

September 7, 2008
Knuckle Sighting

I noticed it this morning. There, lurking just below my finger, is the beginning of a knuckle. Really.

Mostly, I'm thinking about my Breasty Business, as you will see by the following. I think this surgery, although much lower impact, brought up an echo of the past year. I'm sure there will be more that surfaces, but what follows is what has been mined from my current musings and conversations.

The Year Revisited

It has recently come to light that each of my daughters was holding a lot of emotion about this past year, that each was dealing with it in her own way, with her own supports. This should not be news, but it makes me realize that I was maintaining a bit of a double standard. I wanted so much to carry on with life as usual, and we did in many ways; but it was not life as usual, and it was not really fair to expect it to seem that way. The biggest revelation is that we were all trying to protect each other from overload at various times. I am trying to swallow this and appreciate that it probably could not have been any other way.

It does make sense, and helps another puzzle piece fall into place, to learn that each girl, and Duke, too, had other people to talk to and cry with. In the end, I am glad that there were supports for each one of them. They did not want me to feel badly about seeing them hurt, or take it on myself that I was causing it. But it is important for me to know about it, to be aware of how they were feeling. It helps me feel more connected to them.

Somewhere in there, I was wondering how they were doing. People would ask me how they were, and I would reply that they seemed to be doing fine. Kate and Gale's experience of breast cancer is more that people are treated and are then fine afterwards. This is obviously only part of the story, and how could it be otherwise? I had missed the part when they were upset and scared. Other people had helped them with it.

It is the most difficult thing that I could not be the one to comfort my own children, that I had given up that part of being a mother. I am now understanding and letting it in that they could not bear for me to have to endure more load than I already was. We were open with the girls about what was happening during each step of the way, filling them in on the information, the choices, and how we felt. But I realize that there were times that I was teary when they were not around. Sometimes it was Duke's shoulder that was rained on. I said then, and still say, that most of my tears came from people's kindnesses and help. Perhaps this was partially an outlet for all the other emotions rattling around.

Either way, I am grateful to know now what was going on for the girls, and that it now feels safe to fill me in. I couldn't have expressed that this was missing, but I knew that something was not right.

For each of the girls there was a different time period that was more difficult. Gale picked up on my being a little "off" during chemotherapy. I was aware that during the first week following each treatment, particularly the first four, it took tremendous energy to deal with the fatigue and nausea. Even though I was never bedridden, even though I tried to do as much as possible, I still was much more inward than I typically am. It took a lot of focus to keep as even as I was, and so I had less energy for anything or anyone else. As much as I tried to compensate for this, it would have been impossible to do so completely, and Gale picked up on my less-than-complete presence. I was glad that she was able to talk with a friend whose mother had gone through some of the same treatment.

Kate's more challenging time was right in the beginning when we learned of the diagnosis and for the several weeks following, when information kept unfolding about the ensuing treatment. She was away at camp during two of those weeks, including the surgery for the hematoma evacuation following the lumpectomy. This was actually in some ways an excellent place for her to be, since camp is one of the places she receives the most support, and feels free to cry, laugh, and be totally herself.

She felt that the atmosphere in the house was heavy until my birthday party in the beginning of August last year. Certainly, we were reeling from the whole thing, and although I didn't experience the party as a turning point in the same way that she did, it was around this time that the treatment plan fell into place, so it really was like taking a deep breath before moving forward.

I can't emphasize enough the importance of community throughout this time. It was different people at different times in different ways, but it all matters. Each message, each morsel of food, each card or phone call, each positive vibe that was broadcast all contributed to my being able to bounce back that much more quickly, to rebound and get back on track.

Two days after my most recent surgery I am feeling well and have a lot of energy. Even yesterday, I went to the town fair with Kate and her friend, and we walked home, which is probably close to two miles. I was a little tired when we got back, but with a little downtime, it was fun to go to Kate's soccer game in the afternoon. I have been on Tylenol and Advil since yesterday morning, and I think this is helping the rest of my system to feel better. We are one step closer to putting it all behind us, and the relief from that is immense. We could not have known how big it would be until experiencing it.

September 14, 2008
Green Light, Red Light

I have been cleared by Hand Man and Plastic Guy to ride my bike. Handy Man looked at the new x-ray and noticed that the bone had compressed a bit.

"That's okay," he said. "It should do that."

We still don't see a lot of bone growth, but it could be there and we're not seeing it yet.

"Your hand went through a lot," he added. He went on to say again that if I was a teenager, it would be further along. If he says that one more time, I will obviously have to bop him one (like a teeny bopper?) and remind him that despite my best efforts, I am not, in fact a teenager, and my bone growth will reflect that. I'm doing my best here.

I was having a little trouble discerning the progress, and so I said, "So you don't hate it?"

He paused for just a fraction before replying "Right. I don't hate it. In fact, you're further along than I thought you would be. Let's bump our next appointment out six weeks. We still may decide at some point that it's not healing enough, but for now let's start some strength training in it and see how it goes."

Not exactly a ringing endorsement, but I'll take it and keep hoping for the best.

I asked about biking. "Isn't that what got you into this mess in the first place?" I nodded enthusiastically. "So you want to get back on the horse?" There may be a place for a horse in this metaphor, but it would be me chomping at the bit, not me overcoming my fear about riding again.

"It's a source of tremendous fun and a stress reliever for me," I tell him.

The weather has not cooperated with this venture, and I'm realizing that my shoulder is incredibly stiff after trying to not use my arm for a week, so we'll see. It's very frustrating.

My visit with Plastic Guy was brief. The nurse removed the butterfly steri-strips while we talked about What Next. As previously noted, it will likely be surgery in three months, at the beginning of December. Healing time will be a bit longer than with this past one, but will bring me into greater symmetry if I choose to go that route, which at this point I probably will.

After my initial burst of relief at having energy, I suffered a few days of vexation that I am still not back to myself completely. My hand is still stiff, and I cannot make a fist or open it completely. I have some soreness from the surgery that is easier to ignore in some bras than others. I should do a treatment-related bra rating sometime. Life goes on, bra...

I know that my impatience (or is that the flower?) gets me sometimes, but I get so tired of the many exercises and waiting to do what I want to do. Some form of exercise is clearly my salvation, and when I ignore this, everyone suffers.

My social work license renews on October 1, and I finally wrote to the Licensing Board this week saying, Hey Pals, this has been kind of a freakish year for me, and here's why...do you think I could have a few extra months to get together 30 hours of continuing education credits, especially since I completed two graduate certificates in 2006?

A representative for the Board wrote back on the SAME DAY, and said, Dude, you've been through the medical wringer. Why don't you take two years to do the extra credits (and that way we won't have to do any extra paper work ourselves)?

This was a most generous response, and now I seem to possess the motivation of a slug. I'm going back to my slothenly ways. Maybe just having a wee breather will help me feel a tad more energetic about it. At any rate, I know I'll get to it.

I will see Hugs this week, in addition to my O.T. A mere three appointments, as opposed to the five of this past week. I'm sure there was something else to Babylon about, but it appears to have disappeared behind the call of the Patriots.

Hope things are less humid in your corners of the world.

September 20, 2008
Color Wars

Okay, so now I'm a brunette. I'm sure this has nothing to do with my experience of last weekend when I went to buy movie tickets and the girl asked if I was over 62.

"No," I replied brightly, waiting for change from my twenty.

"Because if you are," she went on, "there's a discount."

I raised my eyebrows and smiled and continued to wait for my change.

She couldn't leave it alone. "You look really young, but I just thought I would ask."

All I could do was keep on smiling and waiting until she handed me the money, but she wasn't done yet.

"I didn't mean to offend you," she continued. "Really."

I smiled in a way that I hoped was reassuring and tried not to evince the strain I felt from resisting my urge to reach through the tiny window and strangle her. Her math skills must have been wanting, because it was just short of an eternity later when she handed through my tickets with the buck.

"I definitely don't want to offend you. Sorry."

Speechless, I raced the hell out of there.

Three days later, I was sitting in the chair discussing my possibilities with my delightful beauty parlor lady. In addition to cleaning up the cut from early June, we settled on the least permanent version of the color my hair used to be, so that it will wash out over a few weeks if I decide to go back to natural. I'm still not sure what I think, as it is a combination of shorter hair and different color. Apart from my family and anyone at the hair salon, no one except the mother of one of my clients commented (and she knows nothing of my Breasty Business). Interesting. I'll try to get a photo out; Duke insisted that I wait until after a shower so that it minimizes the impact of bed head, which I'm now fully capable of displaying.

I saw Hugs this week. He feels I'm doing well on the Tamoxifen, and we will revisit the question of what the best medication is in probably another year or so. At this point, I am still not officially declared postmenopausal. He asks again about my last cycle, which was after the very first round of chemo. He cautions that because I am not OM (officially menopausal), we need to be sure that we're using birth control. He clearly must be reading studies not available to the rest of us that cite chemotherapy and multiple breast surgeries as an aphrodisiac.

I tell him that I'm hoping that the vasectomy is still working for us; I know I have mentioned this before, too. Where are his notes?! So much fun to go over this information again. Our visit is otherwise unremarkable, and the next one will be in the new year, and then they will begin to space a little further apart. He gives me a referral for physical therapy for my shoulder should I want their help with the stiffness and weakness I am experiencing there.

I also received notice of my next surgery. This one will entail a slight reduction of Parton and nipple construction for Dolly. They are not usually so efficient at scheduling, and I am a little taken aback, as I am not feeling completely over this one yet. December 5 feels soon, and I am trying to resist the urge to cancel. If I ultimately decide that I don't want it, I can can it, but probably it makes sense to get it done while I'm still in the mode. No point stretching this thing further out than I need to.

The letter indicated an overnight stay, which I had thought I wouldn't need, but I guess that some people do, and they would rather plan for that than not. I'll take it up with Plastic Guy when I see him. I know that the next surgery is more intrusive than this past one, so I may not go bounding out of the hospital; but I do seem to want to get the hell out of there as soon as possible, so I'm hoping to avoid an overnight. I would rather be woken by my menagerie of furry creatures than the clanging of hospital bells.

Duke has inadvertently let me know that he considered this surgery less strenuous than the others. We were walking on the Sunday after my Friday surgery, having started the uphill in the last mile toward home (so, mile three). I lagged just a little behind, and I brought this up. He retorted that I do that to him all the time; he was clearly forgetting that I was two days post-op and not quite up to jogging.

And last Saturday (so eight days post-op), we went to Kate's soccer game, and I noticed as we got out of the car that he was carrying Frisbees. I do adore Frisbee, and there was certainly a lot of space to play. However, even though it was now a whole week beyond the knife, I wasn't quite up to the usual jumping and twisting. I am heartened by his oversight, because it means that I must not appear too off the mark. Still, I am not quite better.

On the other hand (hee hee), I got on my bike yesterday!! Yeaaaaaa! All I did was toodle a few miles near the house, but it is definitely doable. The hill posed a challenge for my shoulder/chest area, which is a little tricky, but on the flats I'm totally fine. I'll definitely get out later.

My injured hand is coming back slowly. I still can't make a fist or straighten it out, but it's better. I'm amazed by my new O.T. person, who clearly knows each little tendon and ligament and how to help stretch/strengthen it. And I learned something about swelling and scar tissue. Did you know that swelling often produces scar tissue? I didn't. When the fluid comes in, it brings with it little bits and pieces that often get left behind and form scar tissue so that where there is a lot of swelling there is likely to be more scarring.

That means reducing swelling is more than just a comfort thing. Think of a wave that comes in and recedes, leaving behind various amounts of debris. If the wave is locked into a sheet of skin, the debris has nowhere else to go, so it is deposited along the way. This makes me even more unhappy with the surgeon who produced the fluid to begin with. Deep breath. I'm still hoping for full recovery.

It's another stunner of a day. Time to get on it!

September 21, 2008
Positive Cycle

On the Bike!!! Duke and I did the 16-mile loop to the Stow airport and back. So fun. A little sluggish, but all my various parts held up very nicely, so I'm up for more!! Yea!

October 12, 2008
Getting a Grip

This is what I am endeavoring to do. I'm getting there, but as I was receiving change from a store the other day, I couldn't quite close my hot little fist around the coins. I'm not usually one to resist change, but I will have to keep working on it. My last authorized O.T. appointment is this Wednesday, and I will see the Hand Man the following week. We'll see what he has to say.

I'm also thinking about my surgery in December. I'm feeling better and less sore from the last surgery. I've been on my bike a few times for

15-20 miles, and I'm preparing to do a staff training for a very large group. Life is moving on. Am I prepared for this little setback?

It's hard to go there, but it's hard not to if I don't want to revisit this down the line. I signed up for this staged event. There was no way to know what it would be like, or that I would throw in a little hand surgery in the middle of it. I'll see Plastic Guy in a couple of weeks, and we can talk about it then. The idea behind this whole reconstructive adventure was to be able to not think about it all so much, and to be able to wear clothes normally, and I'm not quite there. I don't always vote for symmetry in the general aesthetics department, but in this case I'm in favor.

The timing is probably good in that it's enough before the holidays so that I will be in full party mode by the time Christmas hits (but off my own personal stash of party enhancers), and hopefully ready for the ski slopes by January.

We had a great time visiting Gale at Bennington last weekend. It was a terrific mix of doing some of the college stuff (like listening to Liz Coleman, the president, speak), going to a faculty workshop and student performance in the evening, and just bumming around town and doing our family stuff. Gale (or was it Kate?) described Bennington as a mix between Parker and Rowe, both places that Gale has loved.

She's working hard, and it seems like she has been there for a long time in some ways. We were able to spend a little time with some of her friends there and with Nick on the way back. And we visited Benny, the 4-foot chocolate moose in the chocolate shop in town; one fun thing to the next. Maybe next time we'll go further afield and explore the area. During the one night we stayed in Bennington, Duke and I left Kate to the wilds of campus with Gale while we opted for an overnight in a cozy little motel.

October 23, 2008
Hand Delivered

Free! Saw the Handy Man yesterday, who was very impressed with my progress.

"Excellent," he exclaimed, "particularly considering the complicated nature of your fracture."

He feels that it will likely continue to improve, although even if it didn't, it is still pretty good. I do not quite share his level of enthusiasm, as it still feels stiff to me, and there remains some swelling in my fingers, making it difficult to do some things, like tie my shoes. But my yardstick is my other hand, whereas his is his other patients, some of whom are barely able to move their fingers.

I suppose that some of my desire to get my hand back to normal is driven by the fact that I am already dealing with altered body parts. I am able to do a lot of stuff, although the strength in my hand/arm is definitely much less than in my other arm, or than it was.

I'll keep working on it; I'm wearing Kinesio tape on it (which sounds like I'm sneezing every time I say it). This is the stuff that some of the athletes wore during the Olympics. The beige was most readily available, and I'm just wearing one square, nothing as elaborate as Kerri Walsh (but she is a dandy advertisement for the stuff). They do have a lovely blue, and a pinkish red, and black. I considered my winter couture, and if I were to continue with this stuff I would start to make lovely little collages; but as it is, I have to remind myself to put the stuff on. The idea, in my case, is to help the knot of scar tissue dislodge from anything else (like my tendons) so that I will be able to lift my finger up in the air. So when I say that I am not willing to lift my finger to do something, I mean it literally. I would if I could.

At any rate, I am dismissed from the Hand Man, although he did endorse another month of O.T. We'll see if my insurance company thinks that this is a good idea. I think they will, but I'm not as confident that they will also put their money where their mouth is.

We had Ms. Gale home last weekend. It was great to have her around, however briefly. We're all getting used to communicating in multiple ways (text, e-mail, Skype). It's a world of options, isn't it?

More after the Plastic consult on Friday.

October 26, 2008
Sorting....

I saw Plastic Guy on Friday, along with Tall Gal assistant. They were very nice, as always. I asked a couple of questions, like how come I sometimes feel this rush of warmth in my arm? There is no other symptom associated with it, and no pain, which is what he asked. I think (and he confirmed) that it probably has something to do with the re-wiring of some of my internal stuff. He was not at all concerned. It is just weird and completely unpredictable. It's like blushing, only no one knows but me. Some people get hot under the collar. I stick to the arm.

I also asked whether the upcoming surgery necessitated an overnight stay. He replied that some women are really pleased about having a night Chez Newton-Wellesley or Emerson, but this is not the case for me, so I will be able to go home. The surgery is a little more extensive than the one in September, and he is suggesting that I take a week off work. This bums me out because of all the time I have already taken off, but this whole thing has not exactly been about convenience. It does mean another ride on the Percocet Express. Yikes.

I do not absolutely have to have this surgery. This is not strict medical necessity (although irrationally, part of me will be relieved to have the Other Side looked into, and have the pathology report come back clean). I asked what his recommendation was. He is in favor, as one might expect. This is, after all, what he does for a living. That said, he made it clear that women make all kinds of choices. He referred to one woman who absolutely did not want to do anything else, and another who would not stop until it was all done.

Technical Alert!! You are now at risk for Too Much Information!!!

He asked if I had thought about nipple placement. Apart from trying to avoid places like, say, my elbow or nose, I had not given it a second's thought. He said that there are women who spend hours measuring, of all the odd things. There is no possibility of exact breast duplication, so that can't be a goal, but it is important for some people to get as close as possible.

So what is my goal?

I suppose that from the beginning I have been aiming for ease, most of all. It is already simpler to dress, etc., and having the surgery will, in addition to placing the nipple, slightly reduce (and lift) Parton. I will no longer have to think about adjustments to either side to achieve symmetry. So the quest for least maintenance is more surgery; in order to call the least attention to myself, I have to call a lot of attention at the moment. That oddity is probably the reason I'm struggling here, but I know that once I go through I will not look back.

One of the other factors propelling me forward is my need for resolution, for completion. I feel like I have to see the process through, even if I don't feel like it sometimes. I mean, what sane person would be eager to have another surgery? I knew that this would be a process, and I am nearly done, just not quite.

My ever-present curiosity wants to know how the whole thing will go, so getting this done means I won't have to wonder, years down the line, if I should have tried it. For now, unless something else surfaces, I will once again greet the staff of Outpatient Surgery at 6:30 a.m. on December 5, wish them well by early afternoon, and hope never to grace their halls again.

October 31, 2008
RANT

As some of you may be aware, October is Breast Cancer Awareness Month. While I must cop to humble thanks for the great minds that have done research in this area, and from which I have benefited enormously, I am saturated with friggin' awareness. I have been doing my best to be *less* aware. Everything you see everywhere is pink. While some may find this titillating, I find this attention to be rather titanic in its pervasiveness. Duke was wondering about the soup cans with ribbons. Kate said that she's done, too. Even the finger most affected by my hand break is my pinky.

I say, enough!! What are people supposed to do? Wear caps? Bands on their sleeves? Are people supposed to be starting conversations about their boobs? Or inquiring about their self-exam? My big fear is that some little kid is going to come trick-or-treating dressed up as a pink loop. There it would be, the trick and the treat all rolled up into one.

I actually wrote this a couple of days ago, but in a fit of self-censorship did not send it out. I'm thinking twice and sending it because it is what it is. Part of this deal (at least for me) is the impatience with all this focus.

It's now Halloween, and we're on the cusp of expecting the small drift of trick-or-treaters who will venture down our long driveway. Even with our carved pumpkins, we don't get a lot. It was last year on this day that our Taurus coughed its final spasm and died just up the road. I helped Gale, dressed in her homemade Superwoman outfit (pink spandex tights and a green towel for a cape) push it off to the side of the road. This year, Kate is going as Superman with her friends, Spiderman and Batman. I do love the creativity involved in this holiday. It has brought out the best in Duke as he helped the girls craft inanimate objects as costumes: camera, sunglasses, pineapple, Hershey bar, each of them life size. So fun!

May your Treats be always larger than your Tricks (unless you're the one playing the trick...).

October 31, 2008
Sweet

By the way of treat for me the other day, I found out that I do *not* have to repeat pre-op testing, and my additional O.T. visits were not approved, so I have that many fewer appointments in the coming weeks.

November 11, 2008
Random Update

The next large thing on my personal docket is surgery on December 5.

My hand continues to improve, but incrementally. My buddy Pam asked if I would be all better by Christmas. I know that I won't be, and I'm okay with that. Duke pointed out that my hand is probably at 80-85 percent, which is probably true, and I am using it more and more. Although it's still a bit stiff, I can hold things, and I know that it will keep getting better.

It will take awhile to heal from this next surgery. No drains, I'm told, and no loss of sensation, hopefully (not to say sensational). I don't want to do it, just because I'm a stubborn bastard about not wanting to interrupt my schedule (or challenge my body), but I can't not do it. I know that with my body being the WIP (work in progress) that it is, this is the last major step. I have to see it through.

It will take a concerted effort at times to keep the lessons I've learned at the forefront of my life. I am able to ask for help without turning myself inside out or doing back flips off the porch. There is no going back now to what was. I/we will need to continue to create our lives with all that we have taken in the last year and a half. It is life with an increased awareness of its beauty and fragility, and a desire to continue to live it fully, to live our dreams, and act on what is important.

In a practical sense, I am going to need to shift my view of what I have to do, how many appointments I have scheduled in a week. I'm on the strategic planning committee for Parker and have a bunch of meetings scheduled helping the principal talk with the staff, and I can do that now! It's just not easy to trust that this will be so.

I will hopefully be able to use my post-op week off to ride the Vicodin current and enjoy some downtime. Time to lay in the movies and hope that it's warm enough to walk when I'm up to it (not too much of a challenge; I won't bike in 30-degree weather, but it's no problem to stroll in that).

It is amazing to think that I'm coming to the close of this chapter. Part of the work will be to maintain confidence that the Tamoxifen is ensuring that this is the only chapter of its kind. I will need to find another venue for the written word, or make good on my claim to tackle a book (inanimate objects make easy marks...perfect when on Percocet...).

Anyway, as usual, the blank page beckoned even more than I realized. Thank you for your readitude...(what?!).

More soon, as I consult with the physical therapist on Friday about my shoulder, one more step in the long quest to get all the parts back online as much as possible. Maybe I'll be able to do that sprint triathlon next summer.

November 15, 2008
Don't PT Me

I had my PT evaluation and the conclusion is that I am not to be PT-ed. A spot of empathy, perhaps.

Basically, my shoulder is doing pretty well, especially considering the multiple surgeries this year, but I do have some stiffness and weakness, and she described the exercises that will help with this. She also emphasized that because I'm dealing with irradiated skin, I will need to continue doing the stretching exercises for years, perhaps forever. She said that if I get the flu next month (which I won't because I have just had my flu shot) and miss a few days, the shoulder area will be tight again and will need to be re-loosened up. I just need to be more conscious about the stretching. I'm not really daunted by the task; I will use it as an excuse to do what I need to do to get this thing totally back, whether that means finding a place to swim in the winter, or seeking out Richard Simmons DVDs (aaaaaaaaahhhhh!).

On the way back home, I was pulled over by a cop who claimed that after getting around the road work detail I speeded up past the speed limit (imagine silly me not wanting to dally in the other lane). He backed off a bit when he found out that I live locally (I guess the commuters using the train are Speedos), and then as he studied my license, he noticed that I am a Leo. I've got a cop into astrology?! Then he exclaimed that he has the same birthday as me, returned my license and registration, and sent me on my way. So, the idea is that if you get pulled over, make sure it's a cop who shares your birthday. Twinsies, it's the way to go.

December 1, 2008
Countdown

I suppose I might have been able to anticipate this, but I have become a target audience for all things breast cancer. The other day in the mail I received a reminder from Laser Lady about our appointment next week, along with a request for another referral, a brochure from the Image Center showing off their latest line of natural looking prostheses, a couple of e-mails either asking me to pass something along or to be grateful, and…and…I think that was it for Breasty Business related items on Friday. So fun. Maybe I'm more sensitive because I'm looking at surgery on Friday, but JEEEZ. I will hopefully be a little more generous about this, or at least a little less ornery a little further down the line.

I was reflecting on the brochure yesterday while watching the Pats have their fun in the driving rain, and I confess to a bizarre image of vendors going up and down the aisles tossing packages to fans shouting

Prostheses Heah, get your Prostheses, support your team…yes, and all this before the introduction of the next round of pain busters.

Hope you all had a lovely Thanksgiving. It remains my favorite holiday, and this year was no exception.

December 6, 2008
HOME FREE!!

Duke thought I was out of my mind when I told him yesterday that my plan was to be home by three. In fact, we could have been home at 12:30, but we stopped at CVS to stock up on my various state-alterers and antibiotics, so we didn't actually touch base until closer to 1:15. Excellent!

I'm still reeling on local anesthetic (although they did give it to me in Concord, is that still local, or just loco?) and of course your favorite and mine, Percocet, so I'm zippy zippy zippy, or at least looparoo. Plastic Guy gave me prescriptions for Percocet and Vicodin, with the instructions to not take them both at once. Where's his sense of sport?

He asked again about nipple placement, and we did rule out knee, shoulder, etc., and then he proceeded to draw an entire first down play on my chest. I didn't look, because sometimes these visuals are better left not visualized, but he reported to Duke that it all went well, and that my right side would be more sore than the left. Parton should have been careful about what she wished for in terms of involvement in this whole Breasty Business. This is her day.

When we got to the hospital at 6:30 a.m., there was someone outside the check-in area who I saw fit to redirect, since he seemed lost. That should have been my first clue about it being way too familiar. We walked in and the first nurse we saw commented on how familiar we look. Unfortunately, this was all too true. She's actually my favorite nurse, and was from my very first surgery back in July '07. Duke had been jogging along to keep up with me (being weighted down by computer, papers, books, etc.) and we had burst through the doors chuckling about this. It does seem to throw them off a little to have people laughing at 6:30 a.m.

I'm grateful that they now give you a little Novocain before starting the IV, because the first nurse spent way too long rooting around in my arm before giving up and calling in another nurse who seems to have a knack for it. This one got it first shot (so to speak). Before long, I was going for a ride into the OR.

And then I was surfacing in the recovery room 2½ hours later. Gingerale, the cutest blueberry muffin, and two coffees later, and I was in post-op. I streaked by the nurses' station (not that kind of streaking, although with those johnnies, you never know) on my way back from the bathroom, and pretty soon they were bringing me my clothes. The only reason to stay longer was that Ana would not be coming home with us, and I didn't get much of a visit at the hospital. It's weird to think that I was there for several hours, but I have only consciousness of the first one and the last. The black hole of general anesthesia is freaky. And not restful, I have decided. It is not, in fact, like a deep sleep.

Anyway, I am thrilled to be on the flip side (although Kate is much more accomplished in the flip department after her years at gymnastics), and looking forward to my first movie of the day. My "post-surgical garment" is corseted onto me with an ace bandage that is wrapped fully around my torso. I feel very Victorian and have excellent posture, even if breathing is a tad of a challenge. Like the rest of this deal, though, it is there to keep me comfortable, and is very temporary.

Bobcat has just come to assist, which means that I cannot see the screen, so the typos could get really interesting. I'll sign off for now as he is purring in anticipation, and I'm sure that my babblemania will surface again later.

Your good thoughts surely carried me through the morning, and will continue to float my spirits indefinitely. How can I possibly thank you enough?

December 7, 2008
Breathless in Littleton

So, I think I've figured out that Percocet sometimes has a contradictory effect on me: I get chatty and zippy. Imagine. Yesterday we walked our 3-mile loopy. I did have to work a little to keep up with Charlie (Mr. Dog, by his other name) and Duke, but it felt great to be out. It's snowing lightly today, and although I do love the snow, I'm not quite as inspired to go jogging around.

I'm anticipating the Great Unwrap. I have an ace bandage that makes Mummy an appropriate title for Kate to call me. Inhaling is a luxury that I recall from my not too distant past. I'm imagining Duke holding one end, and then my doing a twirling dance move that will leave the bandage dangling from his arm in a spiral of beige. When will they make this stuff in pretty colors? I know that what I find underneath will be more swollen and bruised than the final answer, but it makes me gulp a little to consider it.

The pain hasn't been too bad; I'm trying to mix in Tylenol so that I can capture the coherent thoughts that whiz through my mind and maybe even finish a whole movie. I'm waiting for the Day 3 kick-in-the-ass. What form will it take? Will it be the emotional roller coaster? The physical exhaustion? Some variant of which I am unaware? Probably.

My digestive system, which went on strike due to the surgery, has decided to re-engage if I promise to keep up with the delightful combination of Kombucha and beautiful breads from Brookline or Acton. Anything to keep it happy. If Tummy ain't happy, ain't nobody happy.

We did book me for a flight to Peru to visit Gale while she is doing a 7-week stint working with kids in Chimbote, a town on the northern coast. I'll drag her away to Machu Picchu, as this is a dream of mine, and I have deemed it to be a post Breasty Business celebratory trip, cost be damned. Ye ha! I only wish that the rest of the fam could be there, but we will earmark places for the next visit.

December 10, 2008
Peek a Boo-Hoo

Like the child who starts to giggle in anticipation of a gentle tickle from her favorite relative, my tears started to flow before we even began the de-mummification process. The unfairness of it, the fact that I did not request this, except, oh yeah, I did make some choices around this, the worries about the unknown flooded to the surface. Duke wore his most patient face. He was taking cues from me and would neither rush this process nor hold me back.

First there was the noting of the huge width of the ace bandage. Although I was sure it must be close to a foot, Duke assured me that in fact in was about six inches. He has an uncanny ability to be accurate about this stuff, partly from experience and partly due to some built-in device, like his sense of direction, which just leads him to the right place.

Then there was the post-surgical garment and then the bandages beneath. I looked enough to know that everyone is present and accounted for, and that there is swelling that Ace is trying to minimize. The stitches are covered by butterfly strips, and the newly constructed nipple is still under wraps, so it was not a very bloody affair, and it is part of the evolution of my personal Wonderland. It was bearable, and with each subsequent time it gets a little easier.

I have been using only Tylenol since Sunday, so I have been able to drive the past few days, and walk (even when it was 23 degrees), but I did realize when I attended the Board meeting last night that part of this recuperation is mental/emotional, and that it is not just about how much physical energy I have. My concentration is not at full mast. I think I will go in to work tomorrow, but just for a few hours, which should be fine.

My appointment on Friday with Plastic Guy will bring the next layer in What to Expect. I'm as ready as I can be. I hope that my connection to the Victorian era will be broken with the removal of my Ace corset. This should help in the breathing department, a highly underrated activity.

In the meantime, I will do a little research on places to stay and transportation in Peru. The couple who leads Gale's program sent me some links of places they have found helpful and safe, a good combination. I have also been forced to aid our economy and secure some holiday items. That's fun.

December 17, 2008
Healing and Feeling

This is the second snow day of the year. Fortunately, it is not a work day for me, so I don't have to feel bad about lounging around. Also fortunately, we still have power, despite the fact that our power line is swinging like a jump rope in our yard (okay, not quite that low, but less than chest height). We are understandably not a priority for the power company. We, with power, look in wonder at the area of the powerless, at devastation resembling a tornado zone.

On our 10-minute ride to a friend's generator-powered birthday party in Harvard on Saturday, the downed trees and sheared-off power poles made us realize in a very small way what natural disasters look like.

I barely slept on Thursday night, as the cracking of branches breaking and falling repeatedly woke me up. The house shook numerous times; at least one of those tremors tore out the Verizon box. It was like being under siege, as you never knew from where, or how strong the cracking was going to be. Should we leave? Go to the basement? It was not until walking around a couple of days later that I realized that for the most part, the branches had been weighted down with ice and fell straight down where they were. Some trees were literally pulled over, and people's cars and houses were hit; but considering the number of branches that are down, the worst part seems to be the power outages, which continue.

Today there actually is snow and ice on the ground, unlike Thursday night's storm, when there were no remaining signs of the weather left by mid-morning. Actually, as the ice started to melt off the branches, the sun was out, and it sounded like a rainstorm as the water poured off the trees.

I had my follow-up appointment with Plastic Guy on Friday, except that it ended up not actually being with him. I saw him as I arrived, but when the nurse came into the exam room, she said that he had been called away to the hospital because they were having trouble staunching the blood of someone who had been hit in the head with a falling tree. What? There was no one in-house who could address this issue?

At any rate, the nurse was perfectly competent to see me. She took out the stitches on one side, checked the ones on the other, and declared that everything looked like it was healing fine. She told me that the swelling should continue to go down. Before she started, she let me know that the created nipple will look tall (not an adjective one usually associates with this body part) because it will compress over time, so it had to start out a little oversized.

I'm glad she warned me. I don't want to put anyone at risk of being knocked out as I swing my body around. It went back under wraps to keep it protected. She showed me how to cut the gauze pads to create a housing for it (thanks for the terminology, Duke). The rest of the stitches should absorb, and she cleared me for showering. Woohoo! The appointment was relatively low impact, and I'll need to return in a couple of weeks to see the surgeon himself.

Healing, I'm reminded, is not linear. The physical aspect does not make any effort to coordinate itself with the emotional or mental aspect. Physically, I am coming around quickly in terms of energy level, pain level, etc. However, upon encountering my first shower in over a week on Saturday, I discovered that I had not been prepared for the emotional impact of my latest surgical adventure. It will take awhile for the bruising to go away, and particularly for the swelling to reduce, which is distorting the result of Plastic Guy's artistry. I know that it will happen, but once again, my patience is tried as it will be several weeks of transforming.

The nurse also let me know that I should take it easy in terms of lifting, etc., in order not to strain the newly stitched areas. Grrr. I need to make sure that I can swim when we get to the warmth of Florida to see Doug, my father-in-law.

My surgery in September had been so low impact; not only did I recover quickly physically, the impact on my body was only positive. I almost immediately felt better, more comfortable, as the larger, more rigid expander was replaced by a slightly smaller, softer implant. So this experience is different, which makes sense since the extent of it is much greater. I just cannot seem to get myself to realize that it does not start in one place and move systematically to another. It goes up, sideways, around, and down in whatever time frame it deems appropriate, and I am not in charge of this. What a circuitous part of the journey is this.

People have said that I must be so relieved to have the last surgery done. I most definitely am, but the end of the surgery just marked the opening of the window of readjustment to another bodily change that is not the result of normal aging. This business of readjustment takes a fair amount of energy. I am trying to refill the well as quickly as I can, but I cannot push it faster than it will go.

Having the busyness of the holiday season is a mixed blessing. It is helpful to have the distraction, but when events pile up on one another, I cannot integrate it all as quickly as I might. Mostly it is what it is, and I'm enjoying each party as it comes up. Party, party!! Today's snow day is a welcome time to regain equilibrium.

From Mark:

Hey Meg,

The ordeal continues. The metaphor of the world crashing down around you is powerful; there is danger everywhere as you navigate through the perils of your surgeries and recoveries, and in your physical world a power line is hanging by a precarious thread.

There is no comparison between cancer surgery and joint replacement. Mine was just carpentry, but I do remember that the emotional intensity of preparing for and getting through the surgery was a completely different state of mind, and did not prepare me for what followed: the simple reality of living as a different construct. I was the same person but not the same. Surgically altered, repaired, but as with all repairs, no longer the original. It has had an effect on my sense of mortality that is subtle but profound. My limitations are now defined, less pliable with fantasy and denial than before.

It does take adjustment. And this adjustment—which can be dark sometimes—occurs when everyone is so relieved at your return to wellness that it makes the inner darkness even more disconnecting, contrary to what everyone sees. This is tricky, being on different trajectories. Good you are writing.

So, surgery done. Hooray! But still more work to do.

As you say, the healing is not linear at all, but it is so far superior to the alternative, and the mind and body are amazing at it. Hope is a powerful tonic and being surrounded by loved ones is the greatest doctor. I am still getting used to having someone ask me, with sincerity, how I am doing.

Keep writing. You help us all.

Love,
Mark

December 17, 2008
Nipple, Nipple, Nipple

This is what Duke discovered on my back sometime in the middle of last week, in the form of the electrodes used for the EKG during surgery (I think.) I have had these leads left on me inadvertently before, and I know that this harmless thing happens all the time. It just made me think again about that discussion with Plastic Guy about placement: it's all about location, location, location. I had been wondering why I crackled so much when getting up in the middle of the night to pee. I chalked it up to really loud static and didn't think about it too much in my groggy state. By morning, I'd forget about it; there was no incentive to look, let alone gain access to my back much of the time. Just another wave.

December 2008

When I showed Duke my latest surgery, he sat studying it for a moment. He was looking intently, with curiosity, taking it in.

"Interesting," he commented. Not a throwaway interesting; he meant it.

I could not know it until that moment, but this was not what I wanted to hear. I don't know what I was expecting, and this was an honest, and really quite lovely response; but I felt a little like exhibit A, through no fault of Duke's. If I had been thinking that it would be romantic, or hot, or even a little bit sexy, that was silly. Wasn't it? This was not an invitation for anything other than a viewing, right? I did not want to be alone with the changes, and I wanted reassurance that I was not too Frankenstein-esque.

Perhaps the problem was that for some reason I was not able to anticipate this. Logic was not in play in that moment. I was responding to the swelling, the distortion, the oddities. I had underestimated the impact of having each breast be different. As one was moving closer to where it had been, the other was moving away, and this was disconcerting. Now there was one more part of my body that had had more than normal life affecting its appearance.

Even as I knew that both would heal and continue to evolve somewhat, it was an unmistakable reminder of how things had changed irrevocably from the morning to the afternoon on the day of this most recent surgery. And I had chosen it. How could I?

Even at that point I could tell that the work was well done, and that although each was different from where it had started on that morning, that they were, in fact, moving closer in appearance to each other, and that had been the point.

There was no time frame for this, though. No way to predict how I would feel. Would I be able to hold on to my perspective, not dwell on it too much? The challenge was to stay in the moment, to think "there is a soreness that I will need to live with, but it is also temporary." Another adjustment.

From Duke:

My love,

You certainly have developed a knack for stopping me in my tracks.

If I could ever take back a word or moment, that was it. We have never spoken of it. I knew that you were terribly hurt. It was the last thing I ever wanted to do. For the first time since the very beginning of this journey, I was caught off guard.

The part of me that has been able to separate out the actual mechanics of the process and appreciate the difficulties of the task, the skill and artistry that have gone into restoring normalcy to your physicality, is the part that was able to answer in that moment. My emotional side was reeling. Thus the lapse in the very support you needed.

How could I anticipate that it was then that I would experience the measure of the change and the sense of loss you must have been feeling since your first surgery? It is apparent to me now that I had been shielding myself in order to be there completely for you, as it should be. This moment was a selfish lapse. Rather than focusing on the enormous gratitude I have for your healthy recovery, I felt the loss of your body as it was.

I hear in your words that you do not fault me for my response. For that I am grateful. You have a remarkable gift for giving yourself enough time and space to sort through difficult emotions, and this affords you remarkable clarity. But regardless of the time you need to allow, you always return to complete the process. I am truly sorry I could not be your hero in that moment.

I will always adore you. It is your heart and soul I embrace, but don't doubt my desire for you for a moment.

Love, D

January 2, 2009
Happy Nude Year

Okay, just from the waist up. Saw Plastic Guy today, who examined the surgeries and let me know that it will take several months (*several months!!*) for everything to settle down and for me to really know where it is and how I feel about it. This means continuing with the gauze housing, etc. The slightly reduced side will continue to settle out in size and shape. Not good for my patience, but important for me to know lest I jump the gun. Not that I'm in a hurry to do anything about it.

He promised that a very small surgery could be the last correction, but I'm hoping that wherever it is in a few months, I will not want more surgery to correct anything. It was funny; as I was changing into my robe, he knocked and started to walk in, and then immediately backed out and apologized once he realized that I was not fully changed yet. It seemed ridiculous at the time, since five minutes later he was taking the series-of-three mug shots of my chest (front, side, other side) but I appreciate that he makes the distinction between my changing time and the exam time. It feels respectful somehow, regardless of how cavalier or casual he may otherwise appear.

It is an odd relationship between surgeon and patient, which I mentioned to him. There is a considerable amount of time that is spent with the patient being unnaturally quiet and inert while revealing his or her most private body parts. It is odd being aware only later. The surgeons must separate it out somehow, too. They must remain casual, accustomed to the whole thing, while for the patient it is this bizarre experience. It is good that because they do it every day and it's routine, it lends some air of acceptance and normality to something that clearly is not. They have to be sensitive to our feelings and aware of what is weird, while maintaining a distance and conveying some sense of confidence about how things will go and their ability to handle the eventualities. Tricky.

I guess in the OR they really focus on parts; they need not relate to the person as a whole. The challenge is to shift back and forth between two completely different modes. Some do this better than others, but being able to do both makes them better at each. They can be clearer about what someone needs/wants/is ready for if they're able to listen when they're talking to her. And the better a surgeon can communicate, the easier time the patient has in making choices and in adjusting to what is happening.

Anyway, I'm okayed for full activity level (although he advised against marathons). He said he would back me if I wanted an excuse to avoid shoveling, but in fact I want his backing to be able to shovel! I actually did shovel with Kate after this last measly 6-inch storm, and it was fine. I resisted during the marathon 2-footer of the other weekend. Now I just have to listen to my body to make sure that I don't overdo it. My family needs to adjust to not being too protective. They will need to trust that I'm not going to unnecessarily tax myself (or I'll need a stimulus package).

Next week brings visits with Hugs, Laser Lady, and the Travel Doc, all on the same day. Too fun.

There's more kicking around in there, but I'll stop for now. I need to choose a point to stop these transmissions. I suppose it's kind of arbitrary. There isn't really a natural stopping place; my visits are starting to slow down and will continue to space out (like me), and I need to choose an endpoint. Maybe after my trip to Peru, where I can Peruse my choices.

Have a good weekend. We are emerging from the sub-Arctic temps, which is great. Now I can turn my attention to things like skiing.

January 10, 2009
Well Appointed (Again)

I had the triple header doctor appointments yesterday. They started off with Laser Lady, who I had scheduled to be right before Hugs. She was a little late, and hurried past me as she came in, carrying her shoes and coat. She glanced at me, and I smiled.

She smiled back, hurried on, then turned around and said, "Oh! I almost didn't recognize you! Hello! I'll be with you in a minute."

She was quite impressed with my "result" which is the term often used for surgical reconstruction. She was the first professional to see it other than Plastic Guy and his nurse. "Wow," she commented. "This looks really good. Not only very close in size and shape, but also healthy. No complications or infections. This is great."

"He told me that he could tweak it in either size or shape, but I really think that I'm not going to want or need it. I am quite finished with this whole surgical deal."

"You know," she responded, "these guys are perfectionists. I have had almost every patient tell me that her surgeon wanted to do something else to improve the result."

"Some level of meticulousness is a desirable thing in a surgeon," I reply. "I fully support that. But I am not looking for perfection here. It is not possible."

I am just grateful that a mere month after the surgery most of my stitches are out, and I am moving from the Frankenstein-esque to the... Hollywood? One more visit six months out, and then we go to yearly.

I raced upstairs to check in with Hugs. He was a little pressed, and I heard him telling the nurse that his schedule is packed today. He asked whether I felt that I was able to resume my life. I told him that I had never stopped living it, but that now that all the surgeries are finished, I'm looking forward to being able to exercise more. He wondered whether I felt I had fully regained my brain after the chemo.

"I think so," I told him. I was never totally out of it, but I was definitely up and down during those months. It took a fair amount of energy to maintain as much as I did. In the year following the chemo there were four surgeries and six weeks of radiation; so, although I may have come around from the chemo, I was just a wee tad distracted by my other medical adventures, if you know what I mean.

Then he asked when my last period was. Again. Isn't he writing this stuff down?? I battled with myself, and used a huge amount of restraint not to shout at him, "AFTER MY LAST SENTENCE, DUDE!!" Duke asked me why I didn't just say it. I suppose I was trying not to take more time than I needed there, but next time I really should not censor myself. Then he went through his spiel again about birth control.

When I told him we were still counting on that vasectomy he did say, "Oh, you have told me that, haven't you."

Pal, try to pay attention here. I don't expect him to remember everything, but that is what pens are for. I mean really. We agreed that I should have a breast MRI, because even though it is not a perfect test, it still gives more info than a traditional mammogram, and given my scattered presentation of the cancer, it makes sense to do it.

After a short hiatus to run to the bank, I set out to find the travel doc. They had given me directions, and I knew the area but could not find the correct address. I ran into one building and asked a receptionist who directed me across the road. The building there didn't match the description I had, so I went into one down the street and asked again. Score!! Turns out they had just changed the numbers of the buildings, so where I was looking for 242, it said 86! Nice. Was there a way I was supposed to divine this tidbit?

I needed a butt-load of injections to prepare for Peru's potential perils. And I do mean a butt-load. One in each cheek, one in my right arm, and I need to go back for the fourth injection because they won't do more than one in each extremity, and not more than four at any one sitting. My left arm is off limits for injections because of all the surgeries, and paucity of lymph nodes. So somehow these three visits have generated yet more appointments in the next couple of weeks. Really, now?

Yesterday was a mini immersion back into my recent past, and at the same time, a reminder that it is indeed past. Laser Lady showed me the picture they have of my newly minted hairless style following Leap Day last year. She thought there should be a before and after picture. Although which would be which, hmmm?

Have a great weekend.

January 23, 2009
Nothing Up My Sleeve

That would be of the compression variety. I stopped by Hugs's office last week on my way down from getting my Tetanus booster (a real shot in the arm). I was just checking to make sure that Roe's suggestion of taking Gingko (an amazingly fun word to say) before my trip to help with the altitude thing would be fine. They wouldn't allow me to simply leave a message. Once I was there, the receptionist was required to get a nurse for me to speak to.

Mary came out, and I explained about my trip to Peru, and she said she would speak to Hugs and call me later that day or in the beginning of this week. I forgot all about it until she called on Tuesday and said that his first suggestion was for me to get a compression sleeve because of my higher risk of lymphedema. Well, we had already established that I would be at much higher risk, like over 12,000 feet. She would fax a script for the sleeve to a place in Acton. When I went to pick it up, I discovered that it cost $60! I chatted with my insurance company, who informed me that they would cover it if I picked it up from a particular supply place.

So I now have my very own beige Size 2 Long (thank you, Monkey Arms) sleeve that I'm sure would make Michael Jackson drool. Maybe I can wear it with my glove and make people wonder what the hell is under there. If I end up with a little time on my hands before I leave (funny joke), I will decorate it somehow. Those fabric paints will come in handy.

At any rate, I am gearing up. The last of my stitches departed the other day, and I realized that not only do I not have any doctor's appointments next week, but I think I have none all of next MONTH!! I can't say for sure, but that's nice to even contemplate. I cleared the dentist out of the way this week, too, and got a haircut that brings me back pretty close to my pre-hair-adventure times. Wowza. It's a weird way to mark progress, but so tangible and measurable; one thing is returning to "normal."

Even got in a ski day this week *and* a walk day *and* Inauguration festivities!! Will wonders never cease.

January 30, 2009
Machu Picchu

> If you do a week-long hike there, it is Macho Picchu.
> If you stay a long time, it is Mucho Picchu.
> If you eat Chinese food there, it is Mushi Picchu.
> If you're from Georgia, it is Machu Peachu.
> If the person from Georgia is making jam, it is Mashu Peachu....

> Think I'm ready to go?

February 11, 2009
Home Base

Buenos noches, todo el mundo! What a great trip, from start to finish, in every way, with the exception of learning about Gale's electronics being lifted. Cusco is built into a hill (a big hill, at 12,000 feet). It's international, which is both fun and a bit surreal. There were girls young and old who were happy to pose in their indigenous dress with a llama for a few soles (Peruvian currency). We took only one such

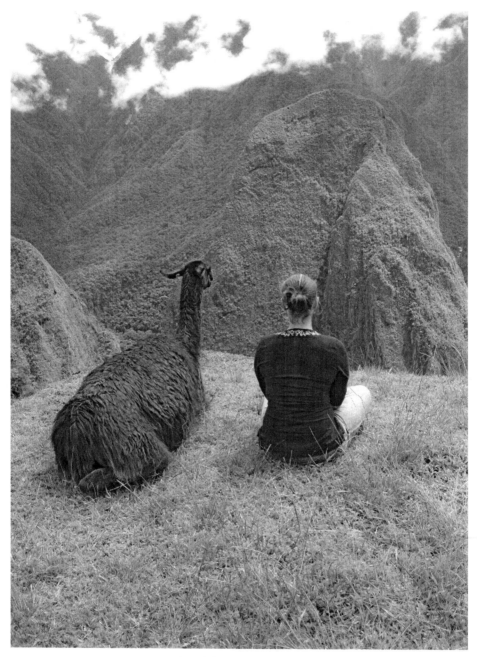

Gale and Llama at Machu Picchu

photo, and the young, young, savvy business girl asked me for change, and was so reassuring about it being fine for her to take five instead of one or two. Isn't that kind? The buck-and-a-half is definitely worth more to her than me, but no one likes to be swindled.

The train ride to Aguas Calientes was amazing as we made our way through dry mountains into the high rain forest. It took four hours to go just over 40 km because we had to stop and switch tracks several times. Aguas Calientes is nestled between the mountains and is a dense conglomeration of hotels, places to eat, and places to sharpen your bargaining skills. Neither Gale nor I was particularly adept at this, though we did improve. We just wanted to give them the asking price, but the merchants expect to discuss it. That's the custom. Any price is just a starting point, a way to converse. If you keep that in mind it doesn't feel so much like you're just being cheap if you offer less. We took a 3-hour round trip walk in the train track (where there was plenty of notice to hop off if the slow moving train approached) to see a waterfall. Those amazing mountains alone were worth the trip.

Machu Picchu is magical, powerful, and a stunning display of what was possible so many years ago. By the way, the first "c" in Picchu is articulated (pronounced pik-chew), because obviously when there, one takes lots of picchus. We climbed up and down those stairs and terraces, first in the rain, then sun, then rain, then sun. The sense of history is palpable, and it is not a stretch to imagine people living there with their sophisticated ideas about how to create drainage, beauty, and a connection to all things. From this perch, you are surrounded by the higher peaks and feel like you're on top of the world. It was a dream fulfilled to go there.

The next day's travel flew us over the Andes back to Lima, and then a 6-hour bus ride up the coast to Chimbote. It is desert 95 percent of the way, such a stark contrast to the green mountains near Machu Picchu. I had not been in such a vast stretch of desert, particularly with the ocean in view part of the time. I loved being on the second story of the double-decker bus (and later realized that the first story had the cushier seats for fancy travel). The movies, meal, and game of bingo were all fun, although I sometimes felt that I was being distracted, as a first-timer, from truly appreciating the extent of the desert. That's probably the idea, but I wanted to really get it.

Gale's Peruvian family met us at the bus, and the five of us squeezed ourselves into a tiny taxi and hurtled home to the first of several lovely meals. It was obvious that Gale's hosts were enjoying her. Their modest home had been opened to share and take care of her. They were so completely accepting of her (as they were of me) and accommodating in terms of mealtimes, or letting her in at 3 a.m. after the Disco. And they were so upset about the theft. It was probably a good thing that Gale was away for a few days immediately after it happened as everyone absorbed this reality.

Chimbote is a large industrial city that serves as a major fishing port, although fortunately for us, the fish factory was largely not in operation this summer. The kids at the camp where Gale was a "professora", for lack of a better word, were charming, open, and engaged. They were interested in whatever was being introduced and appreciative of what gets served up. The other volunteers, both American and Peruvian, comprised Gale's second Peruvian family, and we spent time with them. One of the other volunteers had a birthday on Thursday, and his host family had us all over for cake, cookies, and a humungous piñata. Then we were off to the Disco, where the bathroom signs are either a man standing and peeing, or a woman squatting and peeing. Not big on subtlety there, I guess.

The next afternoon we went sand-boarding, where I earned the questionable distinction of being the oldest person to participate in this activity with them in the 11 years they have been going. I cannot claim a lot of grace in my form, or near enough speed, but damnit, I climbed up that enormous dune and got myself down a few times. Unlike snow-boarding, you can't turn much. You can control speed, but pretty much travel in a straight(ish) line. I would go again in a heartbeat.

Gale's Spanish is terrific, very close to fluent, and she was tickled to learn that one night in Cusco she was talking in her sleep in Spanish!

She was gracious about translating for me; it's frustrating for me to not know more than I do. I can often understand, but sometimes I miss pieces, thus perhaps thinking that we're still talking about giraffes when in fact we've moved on to someone's cousin. Not helpful. And speaking of giraffes, we arrived home one evening to find a dozen middle-aged women in the living room making them out of papier-mache. I have a new fondness for these creatures, which I did not see once while we were there, since they are not exactly indigenous to Peru.

We did see a family of llamas at Machu Picchu, however, and spent a fair amount of time with them at my insistence, observing nursing babies and a mama llama shepherding two little ones as they raced around the terraces. They take their job of keeping the terrace grass short very seriously.

All in all, I arrived home very full, and although it was 24 hours travel to get back, there was no jet lag. I've never been so far away but in the same time zone. I feel that this has truly put a seal on my last 18 months and given me a new marker to reference. I did use my stylin' sleeve both on airplanes and the entire time I was in Cusco, Aguas Calientes or Machu Picchu; it was a little cooler there than in Chimbote, so mostly I was not too stifling. My hand did get kind of puffy in the high altitudes, but that was the worst of it. We were not headachy or sick, just incredibly out of breath going up a flight of stairs. Boy did that make us feel pathetic. Oy, Gale, that's not a whole step up there, is it? Yeah, Mom, do you need an inhaler to get out of bed?

Kate and Duke did just fine, as did the menagerie at the house. I feel energized, ready for spring, and obviously a bit delusional as I look at all the snow. YE HA!!!!!! Life is rollin' on and I am reeling it in. I'm taking a big breath and I am ready. Hasta luego, journey well to all. Cuidate bien.

This really does feel like the door that closes one chapter and opens another. It has been one long loop in life's spiral, and it is time to embrace the new. I have ambitions of getting this journey into print; it feels like part of my way to say thank you to many, and a way to possibly help others who will unfortunately have to travel this road. Not everyone has the advantage of such a rockin' support team, and a book by someone who has been there may help. We'll see. I thank you for your attention, your comments, your humor, food, cards, off-color jokes, and any time you have sent thoughts my way. It has all contributed to what one friend called the new and improved me. I may invoke the Breasty Business distribution list for some other reason, but for now I will hope to be in touch on a more individual basis. Please help me in this endeavor. Forgive me if I am back very shortly with more thoughts that I couldn't hold back. Oh! Or at least a few photos from the trip!!!

Ciao! What better time to sign off with a Heart Full of Love,

Meg

THANKS

I had no idea how meaningful it would be to write this piece of the book. Since for me the entirety of *Topic of Cancer: Riding the Waves of the Big C* is like a long-winded "thank you," it almost seemed redundant to break out a separate section. However, given that I am a strong advocate of feedback in all its forms, it seems only fitting that I would snag this opportunity to acknowledge the many people who have contributed to its creation.

I can't remember exactly when it became clear that the shift from e-mail to book would become a reality, or even that it was something that I wanted. Writing has threaded through my life; from the tiny books I wrote in preschool to the columns that have appeared in a number of papers, it has been an outlet, a means of connection, and creative adventure. It is a way for me to push my personal edge and keep me present.

Certainly my gratitude first and last must go to my immediate family. Duke, Gale, and Kate and the creatures who share our space— Mr. Dog, Bobcat, and Daphne, have endured many hours of personal roller coasterosity and a train of silly jokes. You bought into my notion that life should go on and be lived fully even though it included escapades in the hospital too frequently. Our tacit agreement that we exclude walking on eggshells as a means of existence meant the best kind of support I could imagine.

Without the knowledge, patience, humor, and professionalism of my medical team, this would have been a very different work.

To every person who received the Breasty Business Update, thank you for reading whatever portion you could, whenever you could get to it, whether you responded or not. For those of you who encouraged me to transform it into a book: my dream shimmers because of you.

I bow to my editors, Susan Aiello and Ryan Ruopp and Jennifer Whitney, who helped me believe that this could be consumed by a wider audience, and who helped prune and shape the work into a more finished form. Much appreciation, too, to Karen Kibler who used a keen eye on the final inspection.

Muchas gracias to my team of readers: Duke Stafford, Marge Maurukas, George Demetri, Robin Schoenthaler, Fran Booth, Kate Gilligan, Colleen and Derek Stevens, and Lisa Henry for your early reviews, comments, and edits. My gratitude goes to Nancy Cleary, whose guidance through the publishing process has been cheerful, sage, and informative. My thanks to Kristen Craig who has made collaboration on the website another fascinating learning.

Merci bien to anyone who sent a card, brought food, told a joke, supplied clothing, or carted me to appointments during this circuitous journey. And a special grazzi tanti to all the silent supporters who built a quiet web of love and support around my family and me, buoying us without our even knowing who you are. The world is a better place because of you.

Breinigsville, PA USA
04 February 2011
254842BV00003B/1/P